Pre- and Post-Natal Fitness

A Guide for Fitness Professionals from the American Council on Exercise

By Lenita Anthony

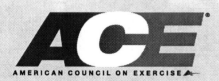

AMERICAN COUNCIL ON EXERCISE

First edition
Copyright © 2002 American Council on Exercise (ACE)
Printed in the United States of America.

ISBN 1-58518-691-0
Library of Congress Control Number: 2001099217

Distributed by:
American Council on Exercise
P.O. Box 910449
San Diego, CA 92191-0449
(858) 279-8227
(858) 279-8064 (FAX)
www.ACEfitness.org

Managing Editor: Daniel Green
Technical Editor: Cedric X. Bryant, Ph.D.
Design & Production: Karen McGuire
Director of Publications: Christine J. Ekeroth
Associate Editor: Lisa Frantz Adlam
Editorial Assistant: Jennifer Schiffer
Index: Bonny McLaughlin
Models: Melanie Ham and Linda Green
Photography: Dennis Dal Covey

Acknowledgments:
Thanks to the entire American Council on Exercise staff for their support and guidance
through the process of creating this manual.

NOTICE

The fitness industry is ever-changing. As new research and clinical experience broaden our knowledge,
changes in programming and standards are required. The authors and the publisher of this work have
checked with sources believed to be reliable in their efforts to provide information that is complete and
generally in accord with the standards accepted at the time of publication. However, in view of the
possibility of human error or changes in industry standards, neither the authors nor the publisher nor
any other party who has been involved in the preparation or publication of this work warrants that the
information contained herein is in every respect accurate or complete, and they are not responsible for
any errors or omissions or the results obtained from the use of such information. Readers are encouraged to confirm the information contained herein with other sources.

Published by:
Healthy Learning
P.O. Box 1828
Monterey, CA 93942
(888) 229-5745
(831) 372-6075 (FAX)
www.healthylearning.com

Ann Cowlin, M.A., is assistant clinical professor, Yale University School of Nursing; movement specialist, Yale University Athletic Department; founder and director of Dancing Thru Pregnancy®, Inc.; author of "Women and Exercise" in Varney's Midwifery; and expert consultant to the US Army Pregnancy and Postpartum Fitness Program. Her textbook, *Women's Fitness Program Development,* will be published by Human Kinetics in spring 2002.

Sara Kooperman, J.D., owner of Sara's City Workout and founder of the MANIA Fitness Instructor Trainer Conventions, is an AVIA athlete. Kooperman was a faculty member for the Kenneth Cooper Institute for Aerobic Research, a lecturer and trainer for the American College of Sports Medicine, and an advisory board member for the Aquatic Exercise Association. She has been a continuing education provider for the Association of Women's Health Obstetric and NeoNatal Nurses (AWHONN), International Childbirth Educators Association (ICEA), AFAA, AEA, and ACE. Kooperman is a licensed attorney and veteran pregnancy exercise instructor at Northwestern Hospital in Chicago.

CONTENTS

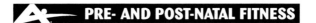

The American Council on Exercise (ACE) is pleased to introduce *Pre- and Post-Natal Fitness,* a guide for fitness professionals. As the industry continues to expand, evolve, and redefine itself, the need for safe, well-designed programs and expert guidance for pregnant women and new mothers has grown as well. The intent of this book is to educate and give guidance to fitness professionals that wish to train pre- and post-natal women. It is also a valuable resource for group fitness instructors that encounter pregnant women and new mothers in their classes. As with all areas of fitness, education is a continual process. ACE recognizes this is a broad subject requiring serious study and we encourage you to use the References and Suggested Reading to further your knowledge.

INTRODUCTION

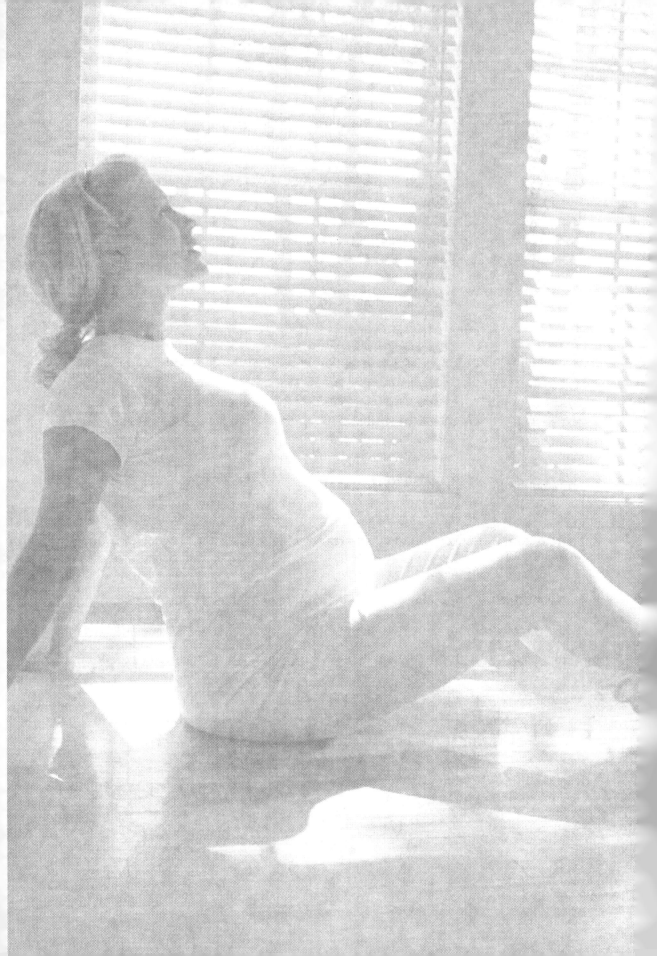

Benefits and Risks of Exercise during Pregnancy

A ttitudes about exercise during pregnancy have changed dramatically over the last 10 to 20 years. The stereotype of pregnancy being a time of "fragility" and "weakness" that necessitates near inactivity has long been discarded. This is largely due to the increasing body of scientific information regarding the safety and benefits of maternal exercise, as well as anecdotal reports by thousands of active women. In fact, cross-sectional surveys have reported that approximately 42% of pregnant women engage in regular activity (Zhang & Savitz, 1996). This is 4% higher than is reported for non-pregnant women of childbearing age.

CHAPTER ONE

1

Armed with increased knowledge regarding the efficacy and safety of pre-natal exercise, most doctors are no longer reluctant to give their patients the "green light." Women, in turn, are recognizing the many positive influences an active lifestyle can have on the pre- and post-natal periods. In fact, it is hard to walk by a magazine rack these days that does not display at least one cover featuring a pregnant woman in form-fitting workout gear extolling the virtues of maintaining a fitness regimen. Conversely, many questions and concerns remain for most expectant women about the specific "do's and don'ts" of exercise during pregnancy.

Are the benefits of exercise during pregnancy really that significant? Are all types of exercise safe for pregnant women? Are there restrictions? Are there special needs during pregnancy that should be addressed in an exercise program? And should every pregnant woman exercise? These are all important questions you need to be able to understand and answer.

The ACOG Guidelines: Clearing up the Confusion

The American College of Obstetricians and Gynecologists (ACOG) first published recommendations on exercise and pregnancy in 1985. This information was widely disseminated to physicians, fitness professionals, and concerned women, who were eager to hear the long-awaited answers to their questions. Due to the limited scientific evidence and lack of outcome data on the topic at that time, the 1985 guidelines were written from a perspective of "first do no harm" and thus were extremely conservative. Specifically, restrictions were placed on the type of exercise performed, duration, and intensity.

However, the guidelines were soon challenged by individuals in the exercise science and fitness communities, as well as by women who had continued to exercise vigorously through their pregnancies with no ill effects. A number of research studies using human subjects were published over the ensuing years, leading to the need for substantial revisions to the original document. In 1994, ACOG published a second set of guidelines. The specific application of these guidelines for pre-natal exercise, as well as the 2002 ACOG guidelines, are discussed in detail in Chapter Five.

Although most of the restrictions outlined in the 1985 ACOG guidelines became "outdated" with the publication of the 1994 guidelines, the use of the earlier document is still widespread among physicians and fitness professionals. You must understand the differences that exist between the three sets of recommendations and the confusion surrounding them. It is likely that, in some cases, pregnant women will have been given information based on the original guidelines published in 1985 that is outdated and unnecessarily restrictive.

While we have much more research today on the effects of exercise and pregnancy than we did in 1985, there are still areas in which the literature is limited. For example, most of the current research involves the effects of cardiovascular exercise, with little data on the effects of strength training during pregnancy. Additionally, current studies using human subjects have utilized a rather homogeneous subject group; the effects on a more diverse sample may impact future results and conclusions. As a fitness professional working with this population, it is important for you to keep an eye toward ongoing research developments and how this information applies to pregnant exercisers.

Benefits of Pre-natal Exercise

Benefits During Pregnancy

The potential benefits of a well-designed pre-natal exercise program are numerous. Pregnant women who exercise can maintain or even increase their cardiovascular fitness, muscular strength, and flexibility. Research has shown that women who exercise during pregnancy experience fewer common pre-natal discomforts such as constipation, swollen extremities, leg cramps, nausea, varicose veins, insomnia, fatigue, back pain, and other orthopedic conditions (Clapp & Little, 1995; Artal, 1992). Exercise can assist in controlling gestational diabetes and help prevent urinary incontinence, pregnancy-induced hyper-tension, diastasis recti, and deep venous thrombosis (Hall & Brody, 1999; Yeo et al., 2000). Additionally, exercise can improve posture and body mechanics, facilitate circulation, reduce pelvic and rectal pressure, and increase energy

levels (Sternfeld et al., 1992). While even very fit women will experience fatigue at some point during their pregnancy, their energy reserve and fatigue "threshold" remain consistently higher than in unfit women. Fit pregnant women also retain a lower resting heart rate, a higher stroke volume, and higher $\dot{V}O_2$max throughout pregnancy and during the post-partum period.

Pregnant women who exercise have a lower incidence of excessive weight gain and are more likely to stay within the range recommended by ACOG. Exercise also helps to stabilize mood states during pregnancy. Active women have been shown to experience fewer feelings of stress, anxiety, insomnia, and depression—negative emotions that are commonly experienced during pregnancy (ACSM, 2000, 1; Goodwin et al., 2000). In general, exercise appears to enhance women's psychological well-being, increase confidence in their changing body image, and decrease feelings of appre-hension about labor and delivery.

Pregnancy is one of the critical "windows" of time in the female lifespan during which positive health-behavior changes are more readily accepted. During pregnancy, many women sense an increased responsibility toward their personal health as they become aware of how what they do impacts the health and well-being of their unborn child. There is frequently an increased motivation to eat more healthfully, stop smoking, and become more physically active. By seizing this oppor-tunity to help pregnant women acquire an exercise

Figure 1
Regular exercise shortens labor by approximately one-third on average.

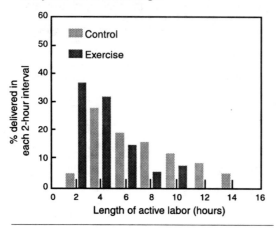

Reprinted, by permission, from J.F. Clapp III, (1998), *Exercising Through Your Pregnancy*, (Champaign, Ill.: Human Kinetics), 94.

"habit," and to realize the benefits this provides, you can set the stage for their activity patterns for the rest of their lives.

Benefits During Labor and Delivery

There are mixed reports on the effects of exercise during pregnancy on the course or outcome of labor and delivery. Some studies show exercise has no effect, yet others show exercise causes either shorter or longer labors. These variances may have been due to differences in exercise programs, data collection, or other methodological discrepancies. A recent study conducted by Clapp (1998) compared the labors of women who continued performing vigorous, weightbearing exercise throughout pregnancy to "physically active" controls. The women who continued weightbearing exercise throughout gestation experienced less problematic deliveries, including a 75% decrease in the need for forceps or cesarean section, a 75% decrease in maternal exhaustion, a 50% decrease in the need for oxytocin (Pitocin — a labor-inducing drug), and a 50% decrease in the need to intervene due to fetal heart-rate abnormalities. Clapp also found exercising women had a significantly higher rate of uncomplicated, spontaneous deliveries and an active labor that was 30% shorter than the controls (Figure 1). However, the women who discontinued exercise mid-pregnancy did not experience these benefits and did not differ significantly from the controls. Another study on exercise and the type of delivery found non-exercising women to be four and a half times more likely to have Caesarean section (Bungum et al., 2000). It appears that for labor and delivery benefits, it is important to encourage pregnant women to continue exercising regularly until they are as near term as possible (barring any medical reasons to the contrary).

Benefits During Recovery

Exercise during pregnancy appears to promote a faster recovery from labor. Women who exercise throughout their pregnancies return to activities of normal daily life 40% faster than less-active controls (Clapp, 1998). It stands to reason that women with higher functional capacities going into the marathon of labor and delivery would be taxed to a lesser degree than women with low functional capacities. Fit women recover faster

Table 1

Benefits of Pre-natal Exercise

Exercise can help decrease or prevent:

Constipation	Back pain	Surgical or medical
Swelling of extremities	Gestational diabetes	interventions in delivery
Leg cramps	Pregnancy-induced	Urinary incontinence
Nausea	hypertension	Postpartum weight retention
Varicose veins	Diastasis recti	Anxiety
Insomnia	Deep venous thrombosis	Depression
Fatigue	Pelvic and rectal pressure	

Exercise can help increase or improve:

Cardiovascular fitness	Circulation
Muscular strength and endurance	Mood states
Functional capacity	Self-esteem
Energy levels during pregnancy	Sense of well-being
Posture and biomechanics	Recovery time

than unfit women because of their greater energy reserves. Others have reported that exercisers retain less weight and score higher on measures of maternal adaptation (Sampselle & Seng, 1999). Exercising women also experience fewer incidences of postpartum depression. Additionally, women who have made exercise part of their lifestyle during pregnancy are more likely to continue exercising after the baby is born than those who did not (Devine et al., 2000).

Ultimately, a healthy placenta that can adequately support the needs of the growing fetus is perhaps the most critical determinant of the advisability and benefits of exercise. Emphasis should be placed on early pre-natal care, healthy lifestyle habits, and optimal pre-natal nutrition to help ensure the growth of a healthy placenta. If the placenta is not functioning optimally, the potential for exercise to place excess and even unhealthy stress on maternal and fetal systems exists.

Contraindications and Risk Factors

Research indicates that healthy women with uncomplicated pregnancies do not need to limit their exercise for fear of adverse effects. There are no reported increases in the rate of spontaneous abortion or rupture, incidence of pre-term labor, fetal distress, or birth abnormalities (ACSM, 2000, 1). Conversely, "extreme" training such as that involved with

Table 2
Absolute Contraindications to Aerobic Exercise During Pregnancy

- Hemodynamically significant heart disease
- Restrictive lung disease
- Incompetent cervix/cerclage
- Multiple gestation at risk for premature labor
- Persistent second- or third-trimester bleeding
- Placenta previa after 26 weeks of gestation
- Premature labor during the current pregnancy
- Ruptured membranes
- Preeclampsia/pregnancy-induced hypertension

Source: Reprinted with permission from American College of Obstetricians and Gynecologists, *Exercise During Pregnancy and the Postpartum Period.* Committee Opinion Number 267, January 2002.

marathons, triathlons, adventure racing, and competitive athletics is not encouraged. While no known adverse effects have been documented in pregnant women participating in competitive athletics, potential risks of fatigue, dehydration, and under-nutrition make them poor candidates for such vigorous activity.

It is important to recognize that ACOG has established that there are some women for whom exercise during pregnancy is absolutely contraindicated, and others for whom the potential benefits associated with exercising may outweigh the risks (ACOG, 2002). As a fitness professional, it is outside of your scope of practice to attempt to diagnose any of the contraindications outlined by ACOG (Tables 2 & 3). Therefore, it is imperative that you perform routine health screening on all clients and that you require a physician's clearance before any pregnant or postpartum woman begins an exercise program. Should you become aware of any of these conditions, exercise should be stopped immediately until the postpartum period, unless the client obtains written permission from a physician to resume. Additionally, it is recommended that you secure an informed consent or waiver of liability prior to participation.

Encourage your clients to give you regular feedback on how they are feeling during and after exercise, and remind them to alert you to the presence of any unusual symptoms. Familiarize yourself and your clients with specific signs or symptoms that may indicate a problem, including the items listed in Tables 4 & 5. Refer women with any of these complaints to their physician for evaluation before continuing any exercise program.

Table 3
Relative Contraindications to Aerobic Exercise During Pregnancy

- Severe anemia
- Unevaluated maternal cardiac arrhythmia
- Chronic bronchitis
- Poorly controlled type 1 diabetes
- Extreme morbid obesity
- Extreme underweight (BMI <12)
- History of extremely sedentary lifestyle
- Intrauterine growth restriction in current pregnancy
- Poorly controlled hypertension
- Orthopedic limitations
- Poorly controlled seizure disorder
- Poorly controlled hyperthyroidism
- Heavy smoker

Source: Reprinted with permission from American College of Obstetricians and Gynecologists, *Exercise During Pregnancy and the Postpartum Period.* Committee Opinion Number 267, January 2002.

Table 4

Reasons to Discontinue
Exercise and Seek Medical Advice

• Any sign of bloody discharge from the vagina

• Any "gush" of fluid from the vagina (premature rupture of membranes)

• Sudden swelling of the ankles, hands, or face (possible preeclampsia)

• Persistent, severe headaches and/or visual disturbances (possible hypertension)

• Unexplained spell of faintness or dizziness

• Swelling, pain, and redness in the calf of one leg (possible phlebitis)

• Elevation of pulse rate or blood pressure that persists after exercise

• Excessive fatigue, palpitations, or chest pain

• Persistent contractions (more than six to eight per hour) that may suggest onset of premature labor

• Unexplained abdominal pain

• Insufficient weight gain [less than 1kg/month (2.2 lbs./month) during last two trimesters]

Source: American College of Sports Medicine. (2000). *ACSM's Guidelines for Exercise Testing and Prescription*, 6th ed. Philadelphia: Lippincott, Williams & Wilkins.

Table 5

Warning Signs to Terminate
Exercise While Pregnant

• Vaginal bleeding

• Dyspnea prior to exertion

• Dizziness

• Headache

• Chest pain

• Muscle weakness

• Calf pain or swelling (need to rule out thrombophlebitis)

• Preterm labor

• Decreased fetal movement

• Amniotic fluid leakage

Source: Reprinted with permission from American College of Obstetricians and Gynecologists, *Exercise During Pregnancy and the Postpartum Period.* Committee Opinion Number 267, January 2002.

High-risk Exercise

Women can continue most activities during their pre-natal period by using common sense and making appropriate modifications. However, they should avoid any activity that has a potential for impact that may cause abdominal trauma. Additionally, exercises involving a high degree of balance or agility (e.g., gymnastics, rock climbing, downhill skiing) are not recommended during pregnancy (Table 6). This is particularly important in the latter trimesters, when changes in a woman's center of gravity put her at increased risk of falling. Women who are not accustomed to exercising at high altitude (e.g., cross-country skiing, hiking) should use caution and exercise at lower-than-normal intensities, as well as ensure adequate oxygenation to avoid undue complications.

Table 6

High-risk Exercises

- Snow and waterskiing
- Rock climbing
- Snowboarding
- Diving
- Scuba diving
- Bungee jumping
- Horseback riding
- Ice-skating/hockey
- Road or mountain cycling
- Vigorous exercise at altitude (non-acclimated women)

Note: Risk of activities requiring balance is relative to maternal weight gain and morphologic changes; some activities may be acceptable early in pregnancy but risky later on.

Physiological Changes Associated with Pregnancy

CHAPTER TWO

Pregnancy has profound effects on almost every physiological system in a woman's body. These physiological alterations occur to support fetal growth and development, while continuing to preserve the mother's normal physiological functioning. The physiological changes in pregnancy that relate most to exercise occur in the cardiovascular, respiratory, endocrine, and musculoskeletal systems. Understanding the physiological interactions of exercise and pregnancy will enable you to design a safe and effective program.

Cardiovascular System

The cardiovascular system shifts into high gear early in pregnancy and works harder and harder until the third trimester. Blood volume expands by 40% to 50% by the middle of the third trimester, and cardiac output increases 30% to 50%, primarily through a 40% increase in stroke volume. Resting heart rate climbs by eight beats per minute in the early weeks of pregnancy and continues to increase to a high of 20 beats above normal by 32 weeks (Clapp, 1998; Hall & Brody, 1999; Anthony, 2000).

There is also a 10% to 20% increase in resting oxygen consumption. The net result of these changes is a decrease in cardiac reserve. Because the heart is working at a higher capacity to pump the increased volume of blood throughout the body and to the fetus, the capacity of the cardiovascular system to adjust to the added demand of exercise is diminished when compared to the non-pregnant state.

The increase in blood volume occurs primarily through expansion of the plasma volume. Accordingly, hemoglobin levels fall during pregnancy. This physiological anemia (sometimes described as "dilutional anemia") results in hemoglobin values 15% below non-pregnant levels. Anemia does not limit oxygen delivery to the organs during pregnancy, due to the compensatory increases occurring in cardiac output. However, during pregnancy, iron stores are increasingly called on to provide hemoglobin for the expanding blood volume, the fetus, and the placenta. Some women may experience symptoms of light-headedness or fatigue early in pregnancy due to mild iron deficiency. Most pregnant women are prescribed iron supplements to prevent iron-deficient anemia.

Hormonal changes during pregnancy cause blood vessels throughout the body to relax and dilate, decreasing total peripheral vascular resistance by 30% (Hall & Brody, 1999). This decrease in vascular resistance results in a decrease in resting blood pressure of 5 to 10 mmHg, despite the increase in blood volume. Early in pregnancy, before blood volume has expanded enough to "fill" the relaxed and expanded vascular space, some women experience a racing pulse or dizziness when getting up quickly from lying or seated positions. This usually resolves as pregnancy progresses and can be prevented by making postural changes more slowly. The decrease in total peripheral resistance and increase in blood volume also increases a pregnant woman's susceptibility to blood pooling in the lower extremities and the development of varicose veins, especially with prolonged standing. Prolonged standing is also known to decrease cardiac output significantly (more than supine exercise). For these reasons, pregnant women should avoid tasks that involve standing motionless. Instead, encourage frequent positional changes and frequent movement or exercise that promotes venous return.

Effects of Cardiovascular Changes on Exercise

Weightbearing activity during pregnancy requires more oxygen due to the increase in body weight, much like hiking with a backpack has a higher oxygen cost than hiking without one. This higher oxygen cost of activity, coupled with the decrease in cardiac reserve, results in a 20% to 25% lower maximal work capacity in pregnant women by the second or third trimester. That means that the intensity necessary for your clients to reach a given percentage of their $\dot{V}O_2$max becomes progressively less as pregnancy advances. Consequently, multiple "levels," or modifications, should be provided for pregnant exercisers.

While resting heart rate predictably increases during pregnancy, the heart-rate response to exercise is not so predictable. It is well known that there is a significant standard of error in predicting target heart rates from age-based formulas in non-pregnant individuals (ACSM, 2000, 1). The additional physiological variables occurring during pregnancy make heart rate even less reliable as a tool to measure exercise intensity. In fact, one study of pregnant women, all exercising at a target heart rate of 140 beats per minute, revealed that actual oxygen consumption varied between subjects from 42% to 73% of $\dot{V}O_2$max (Clapp, 1998). In other words, it cannot be assumed that pregnant women exercising at the same heart rate are working at the same effort level.

The heart-rate response to exercise also changes throughout gestation; it increases early in pregnancy, then falls gradually but continually throughout the latter trimesters (Clapp, 1998). Using a woman's pre-pregnancy target heart rate throughout three trimesters could both underwork and overwork her at various points throughout her pregnancy. Furthermore, no evidence supports the idea that exercising below a specific heart rate reduces the incidence of adverse outcomes for mothers or babies. Fitness and medical professionals should realize that the recommendation to limit pregnant women's heart rates to 140 or less is obsolete. The 1994 ACOG guidelines make no specific recommendations regarding exercise heart rate, instead simply recommending against "exercising to the point of exhaustion." Rating of perceived exertion (Borg scale), or another subjective, symptom-based assessment such as the talk test, is the preferred method for monitoring intensity during pregnancy.

Respiratory System

Pregnancy tends to improve many aspects of lung function. Elevated levels of progesterone released early during pregnancy increase sensitivity to carbon dioxide, which initiates what has been called the "hyperventilation of pregnancy." While not a true state of hyperventilation, this over-breathing causes pregnant women to ventilate 40% to 50% more air per minute. The increased stimulus to breathe improves the gas transport to and from the baby and is accomplished primarily through an increase in tidal volume (the amount of air in each breath). Respiratory rate (number of breaths per minute) changes very little.

Many women feel it is difficult to breathe deeply by the last trimester, largely because the diaphragm—the muscle that separates the chest and abdominal organs—is being pushed farther up into the chest cavity by the enlarging uterus. Pregnant women have to work slightly harder (and use more oxygen) during inspiration to contract the diaphragm and push the uterus downward. This increases the oxygen cost of breathing, which means less oxygen is available for exercise.

Despite the fact that many pregnant women do feel slightly short of breath, maximum breathing capacity during pregnancy is actually maintained at or above pre-conception levels. As the baby grows, most women will experience a flaring out or widening of the ribs and lifting up of the sternum, resulting in an expanse of the ribcage by up to 12 degrees (Kooperman, 1999). These changes in the skeletal system help to accommodate the growing uterus while preserving near optimal lung function.

Effects of Changes in Respiratory System on Exercise

Just as the capacity for ventilation of the lungs does not limit exercise tolerance in healthy, non-pregnant women, neither does it appear to do so during pregnancy. However, both pregnancy and regular exercise influence the oxygen transport system in the ways previously described, enhancing the body's ability to deliver oxygen to the muscle cell.

Hormonal and Metabolic Changes

The endocrine system is responsible for the hormonal changes that occur during pregnancy. Changing levels of estrogen, relaxin, and progesterone have various effects, including growth of uterine and breast tissue, a reduction in smooth muscle tone, and a softening of the ligaments surrounding the joints. This is especially evident in the pelvis and lumbosacral spine. As these hormones are released, a gentle but effective expansion of the pelvis occurs, providing the necessary space for the growing fetus.

Hormonal changes may also cause nausea, vomiting, and changes in gastrointestinal function and appetite, especially during the first trimester. These effects may limit a woman's ability and desire to exercise regularly during that time, but they are generally resolved by the tenth or twelfth week. Many women experiencing mild first trimester nausea find that exercise reduces their symptoms. First trimester fatigue may also limit exercise adherence, and it is important for you to be sensitive to individual differences in exercise tolerance during these early weeks.

Changes in metabolic requirements during pregnancy are also mediated by hormonal changes. A mild insulin resistance causes pregnant women to rely more heavily on fat for their energy supplies, as more of the available carbohydrate is shifted to the fetus. This allows mom's energy requirements to be met, while ensuring an adequate nutrient supply to the fetus. The fetal demand for carbohydrate, coupled with a decreased ability to release stored glucose from the liver, makes less carbohydrate available for exercise and makes pregnant women more prone to hypoglycemia (low blood sugar). Fatigue, lightheadedness, nausea, and headaches are common symptoms of hypoglycemia. A complementary effect of exercise during pregnancy is that it enhances the body's ability to burn fat for fuel at rest and during exercise, thus sparing carbohydrate and helping to maintain more constant blood glucose levels for both mom and baby. Regular exercise also helps to reduce insulin resistance, both in pregnant and non-pregnant women. Exercise, when combined with appropriate weight gain, also helps to prevent or manage gestational diabetes.

The metabolic demands of pregnancy require an average of 300 additional calories per day. Fewer calories are required early in pregnancy, while more are required in the last trimester when the baby is almost to term. The metabolic demands of exercise may add 150 to 250 calories per day to a woman's energy expenditure. It is critical that pregnant women who exercise eat enough high-quality calories to meet the requirements of both exercise and the baby's nutritional needs. Encourage pregnant exercisers to eat small but frequent meals (every two to three hours or so) and to have a snack before every exercise session to avoid a decline in blood glucose.

Musculoskeletal System

The musculoskeletal system undergoes significant changes during pregnancy that bear consideration when designing a pre-natal exercise program. The average weight gain during pregnancy is 27.5 pounds (12.4 kg), but the desirable range for an individual is related to her pre-pregnancy weight. Weight gains of up to 40 pounds (18 kg) are considered normal for underweight women (Hall & Brody, 1999). The influence of this additional weight on the skeleton is coupled with the effects of relaxin and progesterone, hormones that are released to widen the birth canal by increasing ligamentous laxity. This loosening up of the joints decreases joint stability in the hips, pelvis, and lumbosacral spine. As the baby grows and the abdomen enlarges, postural alignment is altered. The pelvis shifts anteriorly, changing the center of gravity and increasing the lordotic curve of the lower back. Late in pregnancy, some women almost appear to be leaning backwards, as they try to offset the forward pull of the belly. Upper-back posture is also affected, as the back must compensate for the increase in lumbar lordosis. The chest and shoulders are pulled forward and inward, increasing the kyphotic curve (rounded shoulders) of the thoracic spine. This is further exaggerated by the increased weight of the breast tissue. Last, as the shoulders become rounded, the head juts forward on the neck. An extreme exaggeration of the vertebral column's normal "S" curve is the result. This is known as kyphotic lordotic postural alignment (Anthony, 2000; Hall & Brody, 1999).

Over time, these postural changes create attendant muscular imbalances. As the abdominal wall is stretched and weakened, the opposing muscles in the low back bear more of the load and are forced to remain in a shortened position. The muscles of the upper back become elongated and weakened, while the anterior muscles of the chest and shoulders may become chronically tight. The muscular activity in the posterior neck is also greatly increased as the head shifts forward. These muscular imbalances should be addressed when selecting exercises (see Chapter Five).

Changes due to laxity and weight gain can also occur in the knees, feet, and ankles. The knees may be slightly hyperextended. Typically, pregnancy induces a drop in the arches and increased pronation of the foot, which may change the biomechanics of the lower kinetic chain. Proper footwear during exercise is essential, and some women may require orthotics for additional support. Pregnancy usually results in a permanent increase in shoe size.

There is some debate over the degree to which relaxin creates this loosening effect in other joints in the body. Much emphasis has been placed on the susceptibility of pregnant women to musculoskeletal injury during exercise due to ligamentous laxity. However, most of the research available at this time does not support any such increase. In fact, some research has actually found pregnant exercisers to have a lower incidence of musculoskeletal injury than non-pregnant exercisers (Clapp, 1998). Increased caution on the part of pregnant women might contribute to this finding. In any case, exercise that helps to build muscular strength and endurance should help to alleviate potential problems by increasing joint stability and decreasing or eliminating hormonally mediated joint laxity.

Fetal Risks: "Can Exercise Harm My Baby?"

CHAPTER THREE

Some pregnant women may have questions regarding the potential risk of exercise for their unborn babies. Being aware of the basis for some of their concerns will help you to give them sound advice and practical suggestions that can minimize any potential risk, clear up potential points of confusion, or reassure the mom-to-be of her baby's safety.

Hyperthermia

Under normal resting conditions, fetal temperature is about 1.0 degree Fahrenheit higher than the mother's. This creates a temperature gradient that allows heat to be transferred from the baby to the mother and then dissipated. Knowing that heavy exercise can increase the body's normal heat production up to 20 times, researchers were initially concerned that it could reverse the temperature gradient and that the baby would be taking on heat from the mother. Since increases in fetal temperature from high fevers during maternal illness in the first trimester have been associated with birth defects, temperature regulation during exercise remains an important concern. However, research has not demonstrated any increase in neural tube defects or any other birth defects in women who exercise vigorously in early pregnancy (ACOG, 1994; Clapp & Little, 1995). In fact, both pregnancy and exercise improve the capacity of women to dissipate heat, and if combined, the effects are additive (Clapp, 1998; ACSM, 2000, 1 & 2). As a result, fit pregnant women are better able to regulate their core temperature than unfit pregnant or non-pregnant women. This increased thermoregulatory efficiency improves as pregnancy advances. One study recording the core temperature of exercising pregnant women revealed that their core temperatures during exercise actually dropped 0.1 degree Celsius per month as they advanced through their pregnancies (Clapp, 1991).

The adaptations that occur during pregnancy that allow women to regulate their body temperature more efficiently are not fully known but include the following factors: 1) Pregnant women have a lower sweating threshold. They will begin to sweat sooner, improving their ability to dissipate heat by evaporation. 2) The 40% to 50% increase in the amount of air they breathe allows them to dissipate 40% to 50% more heat through exhaled air. 3) The 40% to 50% increase in blood volume that occurs during pregnancy allows them to maintain a high level of skin blood flow and improves heat loss from the skin via convection.

Although the physiological adaptations of pregnancy appear to protect the fetus from exercise-associated heat stress, all pre-natal exercisers should be advised to

- Stay well-hydrated; drink 6 to 8 ounces of water for every 15 minutes of exercise.
- Wear loose-fitting, lightweight clothing, and keep skin surface area exposed as much as possible.
- Avoid exercising in hot, humid environments, especially during the first trimester. Pregnant women should refrain from exercising outdoors when the ambient temperature is greater than 80°F (27°C) and, concurrently, the relative humidity exceeds 50 percent.

Carbohydrate Utilization

There has been some concern that because pregnant women utilize carbohydrates at a greater rate, the caloric demand of the muscles during exercise could limit fetal fuel supply of carbohydrates, compromising fetal growth and development. Early studies on female athletes found lower-than-normal birth weights, lending support to this concern. Some research has shown that babies born to women who exercise during their pregnancies are slightly lighter, but they have no difference in length or head circumference. The difference in birth weight was due to a difference in subcutaneous body fat, and at a five-year follow-up, it was not shown to have adversely affected growth and development (Clapp et al., 1998). However, research is still limited and so far has been conducted on a narrow, self-selected population.

Since a well-known effect of exercise is the enhanced ability to burn fat for fuel, many researchers feel that regular exercise and pregnancy are complementary and can protect the fetus by increasing the availability of glucose.

Communicate clearly that exercise during pregnancy is not about weight loss, or restricting weight gain. Occasionally, you may encounter an overweight or obese woman who has been given a weight-gain restriction by her doctor, but weight-gain "goals" should not be the focus of training during pregnancy. Your role is to help the expectant mother create the healthiest environment possible for herself and her baby via good nutrition and appropriate exercise. Encourage pregnant clients to pay special attention to the quality and quantity of their diet, making sure it contains enough high-quality calories to meet the needs of both pregnancy and exercise (pregnancy requires an additional 300 kcal/day; exercise another 150 to 250 kcal/day).

Encourage pre-natal exercisers to follow these basic recommendations:

- Eat a pre-exercise snack of protein and carbohydrates.
- Eat adequate calories to meet the demands of pregnancy and exercise.
- Eat smaller, more frequent meals.
- Avoid dieting; aim for healthy weight gain.

Supine Hypotensive Syndrome

Lying in a supine position during the second and third trimesters of pregnancy may cause the weight of the enlarged uterus to occlude the inferior vena cava. The vena cava is the main blood vessel returning blood to the heart, and if it is compressed by the weight of the uterus, venous return may be compromised. This decrease in venous return to the heart can lead to a decrease in cardiac output, blood pressure, and, ultimately, fetal blood supply and oxygenation. Repeated bouts of fetal hypoxia could affect fetal growth and development. This is called the supine hypotensive syndrome (SHS), or the "vena caval compression syndrome," and understanding it will help you to understand the rationale behind the restrictions on exercise position during pregnancy. It will also help you to decrease the alarm often associated with this condition.

When exercise is performed in the supine position, there is concern that an already reduced cardiac output would be preferentially redistributed to the exercising muscles, away from the uterus and placenta. For these reasons, ACOG recommends against exercising in the supine position after the first trimester (ACOG, 1994; ACOG, 2002).

Some women may experience symptoms during a hypotensive episode that include lightheadedness and dizziness. In these cases, instructing them to roll onto either side will reduce the pressure on the vena cava and improve venous return, and maternal symptoms usually disappear rapidly. Rolling onto the left side creates the greatest increase in cardiac output. There remains some debate as to whether or not maternal symptoms of dizziness truly represent hypotension in all women who experience them, with some reports of the true incidence of SHS as low as 8% in symptomatic individuals (Hall & Brody, 1999). Other researchers feel that supine exercise is safe and that movement of the limbs while supine enhances venous return so that cardiac output is sufficient (Clapp, 1998). However, until there is more clear evidence that they pose no unnecessary risks to the baby, supine exercises should be performed with caution and modified.

Minimizing

Common

Maternal

Conditions

and

Discomforts

CHAPTER FOUR

Round Ligament Pain

The round ligament is a fibro-muscular band that attaches to either side of the uterus and extends downward through the inguinal canal to the labia majora. Its function is to help support the uterus within the pelvic cavity. As the uterus grows, the round ligament may lengthen as much as 9 to 10 inches (23 to 25 cm) due to the increased load it must bear. Round ligament pain is one of the more common complaints you will hear from pre-natal exercisers. If a pregnant woman complains of a dull, pulling sensation in the pelvic region, or a sharp pain that runs diagonally down the lower pelvic region, it is likely the round ligament.

Due to the increased load on this ligament during pregnancy, movements that compound the mechanical stress on it can easily cause irritation. Positions that may exacerbate round ligament pain include extreme stretches over the head, twisting at the waist, sudden turns, kneeling on hands and knees, and sitting up straight from a supine position. A standing, unilateral "hip hike" exercise can help to prevent and relieve round ligament pain. To perform this exercise, have your client elevate one iliac crest by shifting her body weight to the leg of the unaffected side while slowly lifting up the other leg to "unweight" the ligament on the painful side and hold the position for five seconds before releasing. Have her perform three to five repetitions (Figure 2). Other preventive measures include

Figure 2
Standing, unilateral hip hike.
Stand with the hands on the iliac crests, weight distributed evenly on both feet. Shift the weight to the unaffected side, slightly elevating the iliac crest to "unweight" the ligament on the painful side.

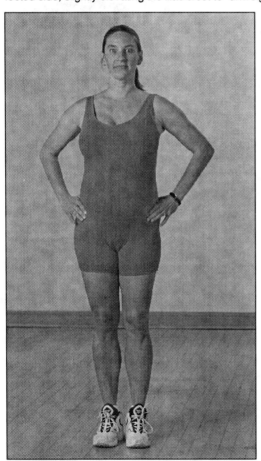
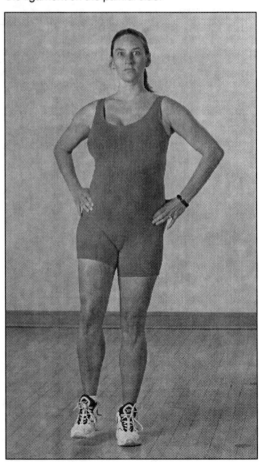

a. Starting position   b. Ending position

the use of a belly-support system, keeping the hips square with the shoulders during lateral movements, and switching to a non-weight-bearing form of exercise like swimming.

Diastasis Recti

A common condition encountered during late pregnancy and immediately postpartum, diastasis recti is the partial or complete separation of the rectus abdominis muscle from the linea alba.

The linea alba is a tendinous fiber that merges the abdominal muscles with the fascia, extending from the xiphoid process to the symphysis pubis. The fibers of the rectus abdominis muscle are designed to shorten and lengthen in a vertical direction (Figure 3). However, pregnancy requires the abdominal wall to expand horizontally. Since the rectus abdominis and linea alba are not particularly elastic in the transverse direction, the linea alba gradually thins and widens, giving way to

Figure 3

Muscles of the abdominal wall, highlighting the rectus abdominis

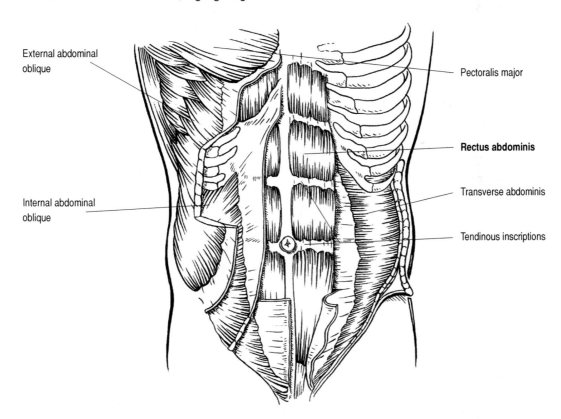

External abdominal oblique

Internal abdominal oblique

Pectoralis major

Rectus abdominis

Transverse abdominis

Tendinous inscriptions

the mechanical stress of an advancing pregnancy.

Relaxin and progesterone also contribute to the occurrence of a diastasis. These hormones encourage a loosening effect on the abdominal fascia and a reduction in the cohesion between the collagen fibers. Other contributing factors include fetus size and number, placenta size, amount of amniotic fluid, number of previous pregnancies, amount of weight gain, length of the torso, and strength of the abdominal muscles. Women with strong abdominal musculature are generally more prepared to resist this condition, since abdominal muscle exercise also increases the strength and elasticity of the linea alba.

Since some separation is normal in almost every pregnancy, it is helpful to evaluate the extent of the gap before recommending, or restricting clients from, specific abdominal exercises. The most common method for checking a diastasis is described below. Though this test is not highly specific because of such variables as the size of the tester's fingers and the location of the separation, it is useful as a general indicator:

1. Have your client place two fingers horizontally directly above and below the umbilicus while lying supine with the knees bent.
2. Ask her to perform a curl-up. If her fingers are able to penetrate the location,

there is a separation (the abdominal muscles can be felt to either side).
3. The degree of the separation is measured according to the number of finger widths that can be placed in the separation. A gap of one to two finger widths is considered "normal."
4. If the separation is greater than three finger widths and the woman is still pregnant, you should be cautious about recommending exercises that directly increase stress on this area.

Exercises that put direct pressure on the linea alba from within, due to uterine resistance, and from without, due to gravitational resistance, should be modified. It is also a good idea to avoid exercises that involve spinal rotation because the internal and external obliques are indirectly attached to the rectus abdominis, and they exert a pull that may widen the gap as they contract and shorten.

In the meantime, there are other good options for maintaining abdominal strength. Abdominal curl-ups can be performed in a semirecumbent position (rather than supine) to decrease the gravitational strain on the linea alba. "Approximating" the rectus abdominis, or bringing the two sides closer together while contracting the muscle, can be accomplished by splinting the abdominal wall. Splinting can be done with crossed arms and hands or a towel, and it is an effective method of

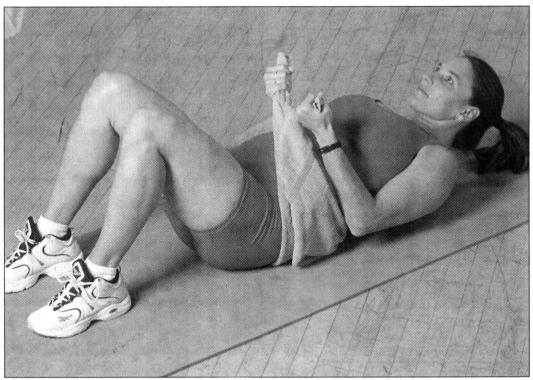

Figure 4
Splinting, shown here using a towel, can provide support to the linea alba while performing crunches.

providing additional support to the linea alba while performing crunches (Figure 4).

Abdominal compression exercises train the deeper transverse abdominis and involve pulling the navel toward the spine while slowly and forcibly exhaling. In non-pregnant women, this creates an abdominal "hollowing," or "scooping out." This hollowing may not be visible during pregnancy, but the muscle action is the same. Pelvic tilts are another great option. Both abdominal compression and pelvic tilts aid in postural alignment and pelvic stability and can

be performed in a variety of positions throughout pregnancy. Standing, sitting, side-lying, and hands-and-knees positions can all be used effectively and are recommended over the supine position after the first trimester due to supine hypotensive syndrome.

Educate your pregnant clients about the importance of trying to maintain neutral pelvis and spinal alignment during all activities, not just abdominal exercises. With the anterior weight gain that is present in late pregnancy, maintaining this neutral position while using the limbs to perform other exercises can provide a substantial challenge to the abdominals.

Diastasis recti is of less concern after delivery than during pregnancy because the internal mechanical stress on the abdominals (the baby) is no longer exerting force against them. However, you should still advise your clients to evaluate their abdominal wall for separation. While there is no documentation of abdominal hernias resulting from postpartum abdominal training (Clapp, 1998), if the gap is two to three fingers or wider, special care and attention to strengthening is warranted. It is also likely that a woman with a diastasis of three fingers lacks the fundamental strength necessary to properly execute a crunch. An appropriate progression is to start by increasing strength and kinesthetic awareness of the pelvic floor (transverse abdominis) and gradually build up to doing abdominal crunches while maintaining the muscle contraction of these deeper muscles. In most postpartum women, these exercises will rapidly improve abdominal tone and close the gap. Encourage your clients to perform these exercises every day, not just the days they train with you, and to focus on using their transverse abdominals throughout their daily activities.

Pubic Pain

The pubic symphysis is the bony junction in what has been referred to as the "vulnerable midline" and is connected by a tendinous seam (Noble, 1995) (Figure 5). As the growing fetus demands more space, the

Figure 5
The pelvis, highlighting the pubic symphysis

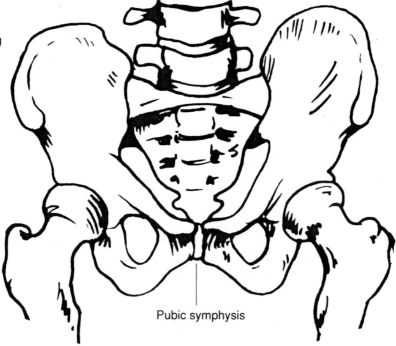

Pubic symphysis

pelvis accommodates by expanding, creating a widening of the pubic symphysis of 4 to 7 mm by the third trimester (Hall & Brody, 1999). Irritation of the joint caused by this increased motion is called symphysitis. High-impact activities may further irritate this joint, as may exercises involving hip abduction or extension. Slideboard training, adduction/abduction machines, and other activities that place stress on this area are not recommended during pregnancy. Instruct clients experiencing pain in this area to limit their range of motion to a level that minimizes or eliminates any discomfort and to reduce the impact level of weightbearing activities. Aquatic exercise and stationary biking are good alternatives. Women should consult their physician if this pain persists, as symphseal separations and complete dislocations can occur. A pelvic belt, which compresses the pelvis and minimizes motion in this area, may be prescribed.

Low-back Pain

Women who exercise during pregnancy experience back pain less often than those who do not (Sternfeld, 1992); however, back pain occurs in approximately 50% of pregnant women (Hummel-Berry, 1990), usually between the fourth and seventh months. Most low-back pain in pregnancy is mechanical in nature and resolves postpartum, but a significant portion (up to 37%) of women may still have serious back pain after delivery (Rath et al., 2000). Exercise can help ease back pain, but it may also aggravate it. Care must be taken to choose a mode of exercise that lessens these symptoms and provides relief. Many women find that when they start having back discomfort in mid- to late-pregnancy, they can no longer perform their primary form of exercise, especially if it is weightbearing. Exercising in water, however, decreases the weightbearing load by 50% to 75%, depending on the depth of immersion (Sanders, 2001). Low- or non-weightbearing activity can help provide relief, while allowing pregnant women to maintain their fitness levels. For this reason, it is wise to "cross train" your pregnant clients by introducing a secondary, non-weight-bearing form of exercise early in pregnancy.

Certain stretches can help relieve back discomfort and should be included in the warm-up and cool-down phases of your classes. Spinal flexion exercises that stretch the overworked and shortened muscles in the low back decrease low-back symptoms in many women (Figures 6 to 9). However, spinal extension exercises have also been shown to decrease back pain in some pregnant women (Rath et al., 2000) (Figures 10 & 11). Pelvic tilts and spinal rotation can also be helpful (Figures 12 & 13). Whichever method reduces symptoms and relieves pain is the one that should be performed. Demonstrate both flexion and extension exercises, and let clients determine what provides the greatest comfort and relief.

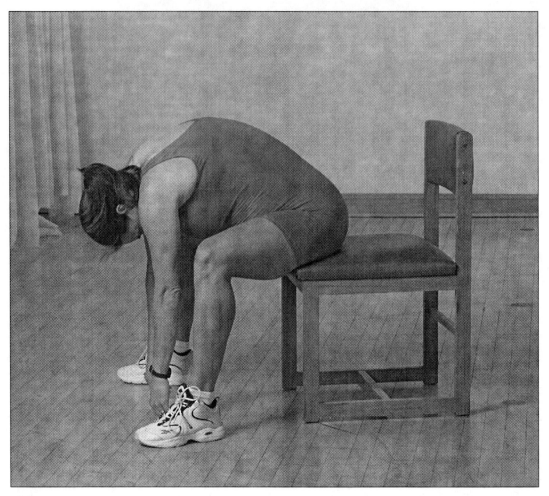

Figure 6a
Spinal flexion, seated.
While sitting forward on a chair with the feet on the ground, move the knees apart and round the
body forward, allowing the trunk to pass between the legs.

Figure 6b
Spinal flexion, standing.
With feet hip-width apart, knees slightly bent, and hands in the fold of the hip joints, inhale and lift the ribs. Then exhale and fold the torso down from the hips.

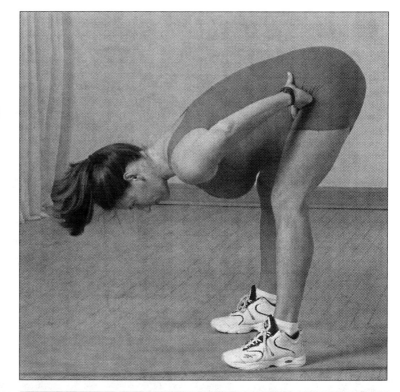

Figure 6c
Spinal flexion, standing.
Bring the hands down to the floor and allow the torso to hang down, making sure the feet are wide enough apart to allow the belly to pass through. Lift the tailbone and straighten the legs until the stretch is felt (if the stretch is too great, place the hands on a step). Hold for several breaths. Return to standing by placing the hands on the thighs, bending the knees, and "unfolding" at the hips with a straight spine.

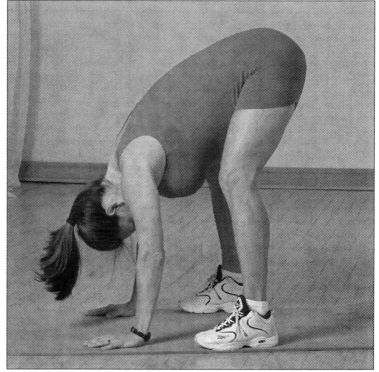

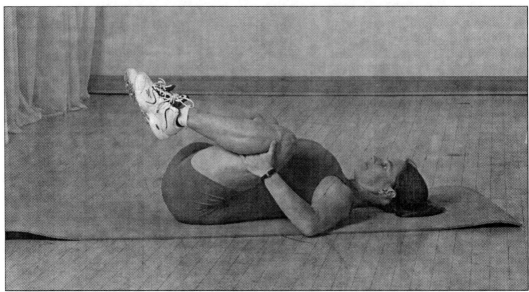

Figure 7
Spinal flexion; supine, double knee to chest. Lying supine with bent knees and feet wider than hip width, reach to the back of the thighs and pull the knees toward the chest with one knee on either side of the belly.

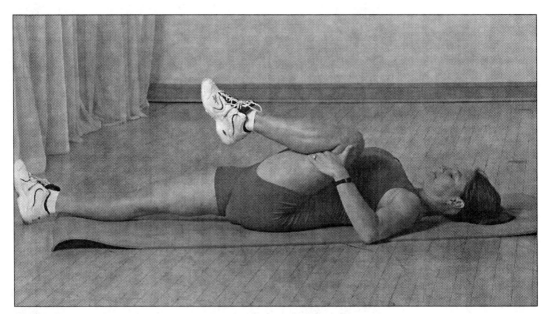

Figure 8
Spinal flexion; supine, single knee to chest. Lying supine, bend one knee and pull it toward the chest, outside the belly. Keep the opposite leg flat and straight.

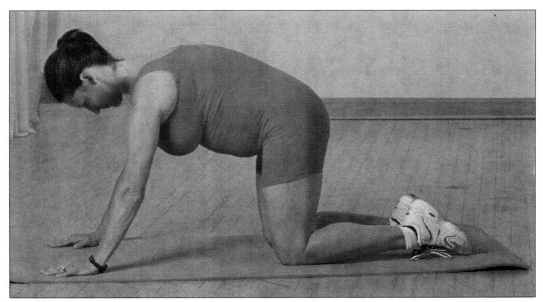

Figure 9
Spinal flexion; cat stretch. Kneeling on all fours with the hands under the shoulders and knees slightly wider than the hips, slowly round the back up, tucking the tailbone under and drawing the navel up toward the spine. If there is wrist discomfort, place a rolled towel under the hands.

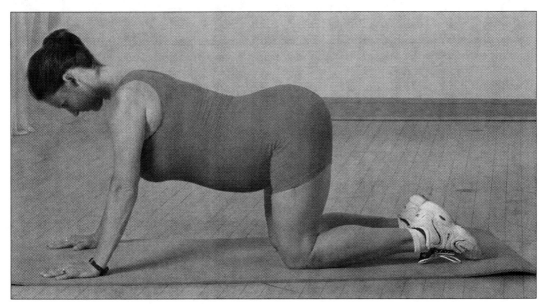

Figure 10
Spinal extension; cow stretch. Kneeling on all fours with the hands under the shoulders and knees slightly wider than the hips, draw the tailbone up, pull the shoulders back, lift the eyes up, and let the low back sink down toward the floor.

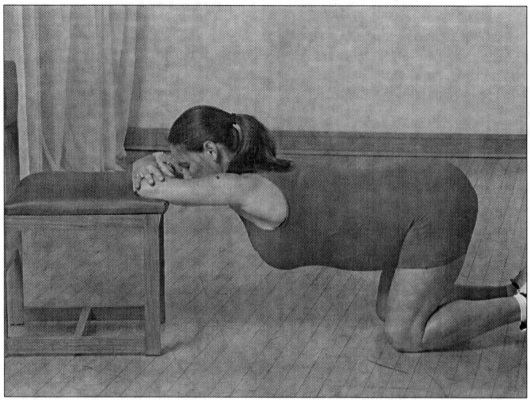

Figure 11
Spinal extension with chair support. Rest the forearms and elbows on a chair while in a kneeling position, allowing the low back to extend and the belly to drop toward the floor.

Figure 12
Pelvic tilt. Lying supine with knees bent, rotate the pelvis posteriorly by drawing the tailbone up and pressing the back down while pulling the abdominal muscles in. Hold for three to five seconds, release, and repeat. The movement is minimal; note the tightening of the abdominal muscles and the reduction in the gap between the low back and the floor. This movement can be done during the first trimester. Because of the discomfort associated with lying supine in the second and third trimesters, limit time to less than three to five minutes.

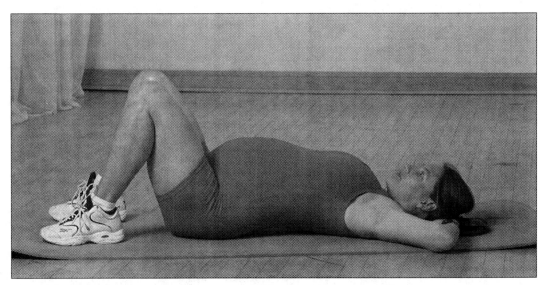

a. Starting position

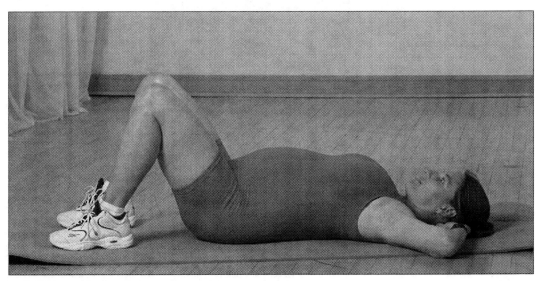

b. Ending position

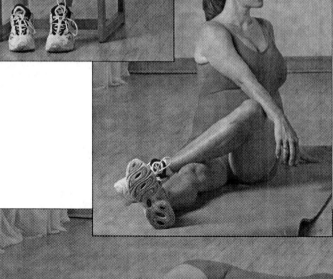

Figure 13
Spinal rotation.

a. Seated in a chair, reach one arm across the belly and grasp the opposite side of the chair. Look over the shoulder while rotating the low- and mid-back.

b. In a seated position with one knee straight and the other bent and crossed over the straight leg, bring the opposite arm to the raised knee, pull it toward the body, and look over that shoulder. (Note: by the third trimester, the size of the belly may make this stretch difficult for some.)

c. Starting from a side-lying position with legs bent and both arms in front of the body, bring the top arm across to the opposite side, allowing the upper-back and shoulders to remain flat on the floor and the lower back to relax and rotate. Allow the muscles of the low back to relax and lengthen.

a.

b.

c.

Leg Cramps

Muscle cramps, especially in the legs, are common during pregnancy. They often occur at night, causing pain that awakens pregnant women and disturbs their sleep. Advise your clients on how to relieve cramps by putting the affected muscle in a stretched position and holding it until the sensation subsides. Teach them the phrase "toes to the nose" to help relieve calf cramps. The natural tendency for most women experiencing the pain of a cramping calf muscle is to tighten it. Instead they need to relax and gently stretch it by keeping the knee straight and by pulling the toes toward the nose. For a foot cramp, recommend dorsiflexing the foot and spreading the toes (Anthony, 2000).

Regular aerobic exercise, adequate hydration, and proper nutrition help to decrease the incidence of muscle cramps during pregnancy. Additionally, advise your clients to avoid high heels, tight shoes, and extreme pointing of their toes. All of these may stimulate muscle cramping. Advise pregnant women to consult with their doctors if cramping is persistent.

Carpal Tunnel Syndrome

Carpal tunnel syndrome is caused by compression of the median nerve in the wrist and results in numbness and tingling in the thumb, index, and middle fingers (Figure 14). It is the most common of several nerve-compression syndromes often encountered during pregnancy. More than 80% of pregnant women have some degree of swelling during pregnancy (Noble, 1995). This fluid retention and swelling (called edema) can decrease the available space in relatively constrained anatomical spaces, causing compression of the nerves.

Exercise that puts the wrist in an extended and loaded position will exacerbate carpal tunnel syndrome. The hands-and-knees, or all-fours, position is one such example. Other aggravators include grasping objects tightly (like dumbbells or tubing) and repetitive flexion/extension of the wrist. Remind pregnant women to keep their wrists in a neutral position as much as possible. Neutral position for the wrist is 10 degrees of extension, with no deviation medially or laterally. If carpal tunnel syndrome is present, select resistance exercises that do not involve tightly gripping weights or bands. The wrists can be kept neutral in the hands-and-knees position by using hexagonal dumbbells (round ones will roll) under the hands and keeping the wrists vertically aligned with the arms.

Remind clients with carpal tunnel syndrome about activities outside of class that may worsen the condition. Examples include repetitive keyboard usage, gardening, needlepoint or knitting, pushing a stroller with

Figure 14
The nerves of the
wrist, highlighting
the median nerve

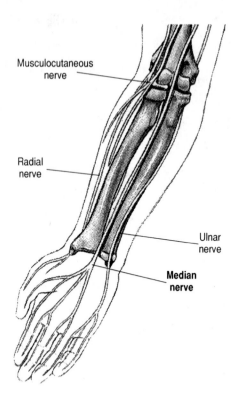

Musculocutaneous
nerve

Radial
nerve

Ulnar
nerve

**Median
nerve**

Source: *Human Anatomy,* 2/e, by Martini/Timmons ©. Reprinted by permission of Pearson Education, Inc., Upper Saddle River, NJ.

flexed wrists, or any activity that involves repetitive use of the wrists and hands.

Varicose Veins

The increase in blood volume that accompanies pregnancy, coupled with the relaxation that occurs in the blood vessels and the growing pressure within the abdomen, make pregnant women more susceptible to varicose veins. Regular exercise helps to prevent varicose veins. Exercise (such as walking) causes a rhythmic contraction of the muscles in the legs that compresses the vascular bed and enhances venous return. This is in sharp contrast with prolonged, motionless standing, during which gravity causes blood to pool in the lower legs, causing thin-walled veins to become distended and prominent. Prolonged sitting can also be harmful. It is best to keep the legs slightly elevated, alternately raise one at a time, flex and extend the ankles, and do range-of-motion exercises. Many pregnant women find aquatic exercise, which can help alleviate varicose veins, to be an extremely comfortable workout option (see Aquatic Exercise, page 56).

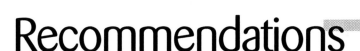
Recommendations for Pre-natal Exercise

CHAPTER FIVE

Exercise Intensity

Recognize that pregnant women differ in their exercise capacity, just as non-pregnant individuals do. There is no "one-size-fits-all" intensity that is appropriate for all pregnant women, and pre-pregnancy fitness level and personal preference will be determining factors. Research has not legitimized the fear that high-intensity exercise is detrimental to mother or baby. In fact, ACOG states: "There are no data to indicate that pregnant women should limit exercise intensity and lower target heart rates because of potential adverse effects" (ACOG, 1994). ACSM recommends that women who are continuing their regular exercise regimen during pregnancy should not exceed pre-pregnancy intensity levels (ACSM, 2000, 1).

So, an athletic woman who enters pregnancy in a highly trained state may be able to continue at a similar intensity for quite some time (ACOG, 1994; ACOG, 2002; Clapp, 1998). Conversely, a deconditioned woman who elects to begin an exercise program upon becoming pregnant will feel challenged by much lower levels of work. Unlike the woman who is accustomed to exercise, she is asking her body to adapt to two new sources of physiological overload at the same time: pregnancy and exercise. The relative intensity for these two very different participants, however, is similar. A pregnant woman should be encouraged to exercise at a level at which she feels comfortable, using rating of perceived exertion (RPE) as a guide. Depending on the individual, an RPE of 5 to 8 on the 10-point scale may be appropriate. Remind pregnant clients that it will take progressively lower levels of work to attain the same RPE as their pregnancy advances.

ACOG recommends that pregnant women "avoid exercise to exhaustion." Remind your pregnant clients to assess how they feel a few hours after exercise as well. Does she feel energized, or unusually fatigued? Her answer provides a useful guide as to what may be an appropriate level of exertion for her. As stated in Chapter Two, heart-rate monitoring is not a reliable indicator of exercise intensity during pregnancy.

Exercise Duration

It is not possible to specify guidelines regarding duration of exercise during pregnancy due to the reciprocal relationship between exercise intensity and duration (Artal, 2000). In the latter trimesters, however, consideration must be given to fetal nutrition and optimal energy balance. Prolonged vigorous exercise requires more calories. The higher the number of calories burned in exercise, the more food the mother must consume to ensure that her diet is compensating adequately and fetal nutrition is not suffering. Eating this amount of food can be difficult, particularly in the third trimester when it becomes uncomfortable to eat large meals due to less space in the stomach, gastroesophageal reflux (heartburn), etc. This is also the period when fetal nutritional needs are at their highest. If the mother's intake is not adequate, fetal birth weight may be negatively affected. In light of these issues, and the difficulty some women have in taking in enough calories, it seems reasonable to discourage cardiovascular workouts longer than 45 to 50 minutes. A typical group exercise class should include a 10- to 15-minute warm-up and cool-down, making total class time approximately one hour.

Exercise Frequency

Pregnant women should exercise three to five times per week, the same as the general population (ACSM, 2000, 1). ACSM states that regular exercise is preferred over intermittent activity for pregnant women, and three times per week is the minimum recommendation. Clapp found that beginning exercise early in pregnancy at a frequency of three to five times per week actually enhanced fetoplacental growth (Clapp et al., 2000). Mid-trimester placental growth rate was faster and birth weights were heavier in babies born to exercising moms.

Some research indicates that exercising no more than three to four times per week may be preferable in late pregnancy. A study of infant birth weights and exercise frequency found that women who exercised five times or more per week, or less than two times per week, after the 34th week of their pregnancy were more likely to have low-birth-weight babies (Campbell & Mottola, 2001).

Muscular Imbalances

While a wide range of fitness levels exists among pregnant women, all will experience certain muscu-loskeletal imbalances at some point in their pregnancy. Postural changes during pregnancy create certain "trained imbalances" between muscle groups that can lead to discomfort, pain, and, in some cases, injury. Incorporate exercises

Table 7

Muscles to Stretch:	Muscles to Strengthen:
Scapula protractors	Scapula retractors
Levator scapula	Lumbar paravertebral
Thoracolumbar area	Gluteus maximus and medius
Hip flexors	
Illiotibial band	Quadriceps
Piriformis	Abdominals
Hamstrings	Pelvic floor
Hip adductors	
Gastrocnemius, soleus	

designed to counterbalance the natural tendency during pregnancy to become either "tight" or "weak" in specific areas. Appropriate exercise selection can help reduce the muscle imbalances that lead to the postural deviations associated with pregnancy (Table 7). Muscles that tend to shorten and tighten include those in the shoulders, chest, low back, hamstrings, and calves. Muscles that tend to lengthen and weaken include those in the upper back, glutes, abdominals, pelvic floor, and quadriceps. When dealing with these imbalances, it is most effective to first relax the tight muscles with mobility and stretching exercises, and then follow with strengthening exercises for the weaker muscles.

Abdominal and Pelvic Floor Exercise

To prevent supine hypotensive syndrome (see Supine Hypotensive Syndrome, page 17), modifications for supine abdominal exercises should be given to women who are past their fourth month of pregnancy.

Short periods of time (60 to 90 seconds) performing abdominal exercise in a supine position interspersed with exercises performed in a side-lying position are unlikely to cause fetal hypoxia. However, if a client reports any feelings of dizziness or discomfort, eliminate all supine work. Multiple abdominal exercises can be performed that avoid back-lying positions, and fitness instructors should be well-acquainted with a wide variety of options. Figures 15 to 19 show various abdominal and pelvic floor exercises.

The rectus abdominis muscle is the focus in most traditional abdominal exercises (e.g., crunches). However, it is important to teach women as early in their pregnancy as possible how to strengthen the deeper transverse abdominis muscle as well. As a woman's belly grows, the stretch on the rectus abdominis muscle places it in a mechanically disadvantaged position for shortening, and strength is compromised. The transverse abdominis, a deeper muscle with fibers that are aligned horizontally, plays a key role in spinal stabilization. Strong transverse abs may also help to minimize diastasis recti (see Diastasis Recti, page 21).

Training the transverse abs is best accomplished by abdominal compression, sometimes called "belly breathing" or "hollowing" (although pregnant women may find the term "hollowing" humorous in the latter trimesters!). This technique should first be taught in isolation, lying supine or seated. Once mastered, it should be incorporated with all other exercises whenever possible. Instruct your pregnant client to take a deep breath in, letting the abdomen expand as the lungs fill, exhale fully while pulling the navel toward the backbone, and then hold the contraction for several seconds and release. You can help a client who is not familiar with this exercise learn how to tense the abdominal area without crunching by cueing her to make a hissing sound, or to say "ha ha ha," while exhaling and drawing in the navel. Another useful cue is to imagine "hugging" the baby with the abdominal muscles, or "lifting" the baby. The transverse abs are assisted by gravity in the supine position, so once a client understands this exercise, you will want her to try it in positions that are slightly more challenging. Sitting with the back against a wall or straight-back bench, squatting against a wall, standing, or getting down on hands and knees are all good options.

Late in pregnancy, women with increased lordosis will find that standing with the pelvis in neutral (iliac crest in same vertical plane as pubic symphysis) is an effective and challenging abdominal exercise. To bring the pelvis into a posterior tilt and engage the abdominal muscles, cue your client to "pull the pubic bone toward the navel." Pelvic tilts can be combined with abdominal compression and performed in the standing, sitting, and side-lying positions, as well as against a wall in a half-squat position. Pelvic tilting throughout the day enhances muscular control, strength, and postural awareness and may have the added benefit of relieving low-back pain caused by fatigue (Hall & Brody, 1999).

Allot equal time to back exercises, especially ones that help to counterbalance the postural changes associated with pregnancy, during the abdominal portion of a training session. Specifically, incorporate stretches for the lower back and strengthening exercises for the upper- and mid-back.

Table 8

General Guidelines for the Pregnant Exerciser

Wear loose, comfortable clothing that facilitates heat loss.

Wear a supportive bra and maternal support belt if needed.

Eat a pre-exercise snack.

Base intensity on perceived exertion (RPE).

Drink water (6 to 8 ounces for every 15 to 20 minutes of activity).

Do not exercise to exhaustion.

Modify exercises that feel awkward or uncomfortable.

Report any unusual discomfort or symptom to your instructor or personal trainer.

Focus on posture and maintaining good alignment.

If exercise results in increased fatigue, decrease intensity or duration.

The Pelvic Floor

The five layers of muscle and fascia attached to the bony ring of the pelvis are commonly referred to as the pelvic floor. The muscles of the pelvic floor have been referred to as a sling, because they extend from the pubic bone to the tailbone and support the internal organs. They also affect bladder, bowel, and sexual function. The weight gain and mechanical stress of the growing uterus affect this area, creating a stretch weakness in the muscles of the pelvic floor. Hormonal influences cause a softening of these tissues that further aggravates the weakness, as does the birth process itself. Maintaining the strength and integrity of these muscles during pregnancy and after delivery is extremely important and can help to prevent urinary stress incontinence, pelvic organ prolapse, pelvic pain from muscle spasm, and misalignments in the hip and sacroiliac joints (Hall & Brody, 1999; Wilder, 1988). A strong, coordinated pelvic floor will also improve control and relaxation during the second stage of labor (pushing phase).

Kegel exercises help to strengthen and protect the muscles of the pelvic floor and are a requisite element of any pre- or post-natal exercise routine (Noble, 1995). Kegel exercises involve contracting and relaxing these muscles and help to increase strength and kinesthetic awareness in this area. Many women experience stress urinary incontinence

Figure 15
Incline crunch with pelvic tilt on the stability ball. Start with the ball in the low- to mid-back, with the body at an incline, and feet resting on the floor and the head resting back in the hands. Exhale while drawing the abdominal muscles in, tucking the tailbone under as in a pelvic tilt, and drawing the lower ribs toward the hips. The neck should remain relaxed.

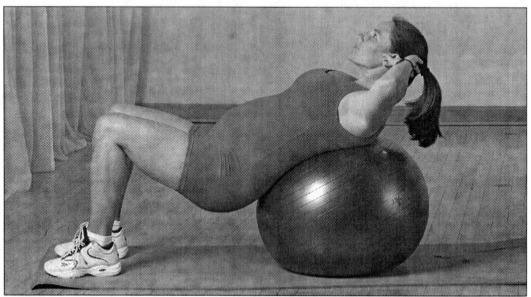

a. Starting position

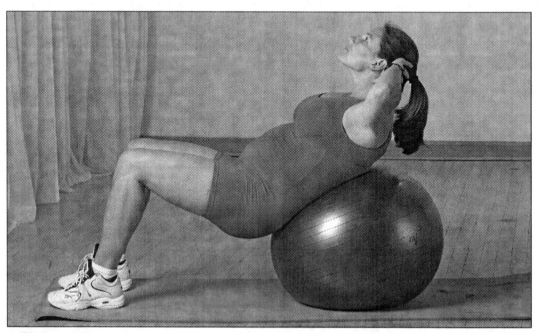

b. Ending position

Figure 16
Abdominal compression. The goal of this exercise is to perform a Kegel exercise (contracting the muscles of the pelvic floor), while contracting the transverse abdominis. To engage the transverse abdominis, exhale while making a "ha ha ha" or coughing sound, drawing the navel in toward the spine as if trying to flatten or hollow the lower abdominals.

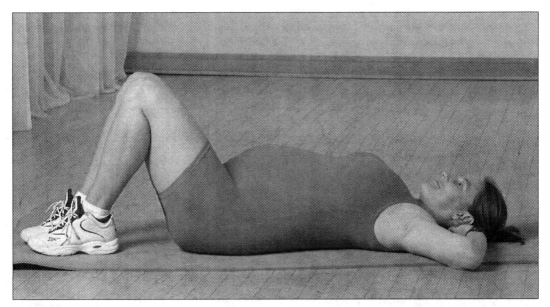

a. Starting position

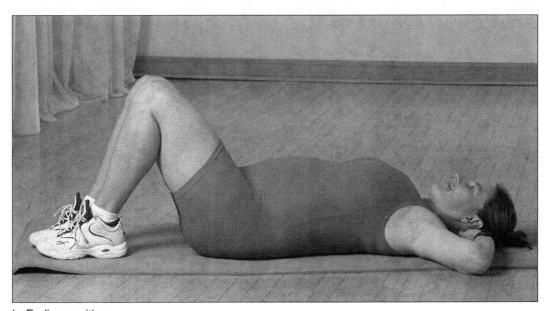

b. Ending position

Figure 17

Quadruped reciprocal reach. In an all-fours position, find neutral spinal alignment (during pregnancy, the weight of the belly will tend create a swayback position and the abdominals must work to stabilize the spine in neutral). While maintaining a co-contraction of the back and abdominal muscles, slowly extend one arm and the opposite leg, hold momentarily, and lower slowly. Do not allow the opposing hip to drop as one leg lifts. Alternate sides. (Note: When teaching this exercise, begin by asking the client to lift only the arm while maintaining neutral alignment. Once this is mastered, have them lift only the leg. Finally, have them try to extend both the arm and the opposing leg together.)

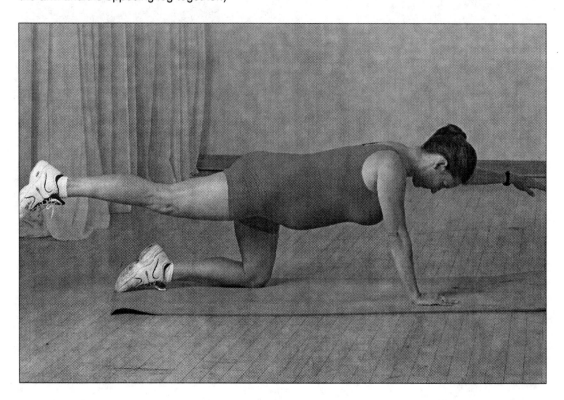

Figure 18
Pelvic tilt on the stability ball. Start with the ball in the low- to mid-back, with the body at an incline and the head supported by the hands. Exhale and draw the tailbone up while pulling the abdominal muscles in and tilting the pelvis posteriorly. (Note: You can cue this as "pull the pubic bone toward the navel.")

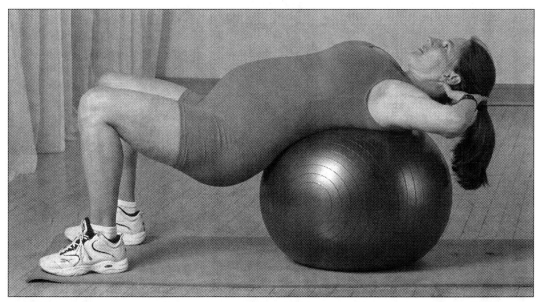

a. Starting position

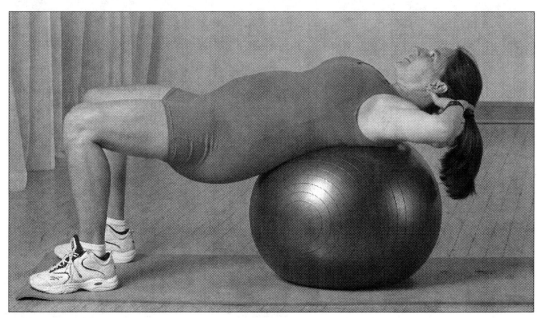

b. Ending position

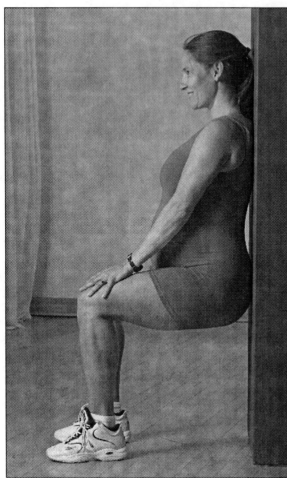

a.

Figure 19
Pelvic tilt and squat against the wall.
a. Standing with the back against a
   wall and the feet about 1½ feet from
   the wall, slide down into a squat
   position.
b. Pull in the abdominal muscles
   (Note: You can cue this as "hug
   your baby with your abs") and try to
   press the low back against the wall
   while exhaling. Hold for three to
   five seconds, release, and then
   return to the standing position.

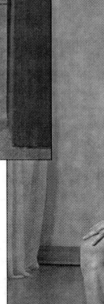

b.

during pregnancy that does not resolve postpartum and limits their ability to participate in various forms of exercise. Pelvic floor exercises decrease stress urinary incontinence during late pregnancy and postpartum, with benefits extending to a follow-up period of one year postpartum (Morkved & Bo, 2000; Sampselle & Seng, 1999).

Teaching Pelvic Floor Exercises

Most women will have trouble initially in identifying and isolating these muscles. Because it is impossible to know if they are performing the exercise correctly, proper cueing is essential. The best cue to facilitate this contraction is to ask your client to tighten the muscles she would use if she was trying to stop urinary flow. "Drawing up the muscles between the legs" is another way to describe it. The easiest position in which to learn the exercise is supine, where the gravitational challenge to the muscles is lessened.

There are numerous routines for performing Kegel exercises. For example, begin with an isometric contraction of the pelvic floor, feeling the muscles lift and tighten. Then, hold for a count of 10, relax for another count of 10, and repeat this for 5 to 10 minutes, three to four times per day. Another exercise is to imagine an elevator going up and down as the pelvic floor is lifted. Stopping the elevator on each floor is a variation that requires more muscle control (Noble, 1995).

Kegels should be introduced independent of other exercises. However, once kinesthetic awareness is established, they can be readily integrated with a variety of abdominal and pelvic stabilization exercises. A good combination to teach is to contract the Kegel with abdominal compression (transverse abdominis). This not only strengthens the pelvic floor, but also teaches proper neuromuscular sequencing for core stability. Encourage participants to perform this exercise not just during training sessions, but on a daily basis.

Relaxation and Stress Management

Most women report that although pregnancy is a happy, exciting time for them, it is also a stressful time. Any major change in one's life, good or bad, can create stress—and having a baby certainly changes one's life! The stress is mental and emotional, as well as physical. Lack of control over circumstances, fear of the unknown, and apprehension over labor and delivery are all feelings that contribute to stress. Most people manifest stress in unnecessarily tensed muscles, from a clenched hand to a tight jaw. Common areas of muscular tension in pregnancy include the forehead, jaw, neck, shoulders, back, and calves.

Exercise can help to alleviate stress during pregnancy, but you can also teach your clients other stress-management techniques as well. The ability to relax and release muscular tension is a skill that will aid in pain management during labor, and in stressful times after the baby arrives. Progressive relaxation, visualization, and breathing techniques can easily be incorporated into the cool-down/stretch portion of any workout. An environment that facilitates relaxation is warm [72° to 78°F (22° to 26°C)], quiet or with soft soothing music, and dimly lit. Mindful exercise, such as yoga and tai-chi, also aids in relaxation and stress management.

Progressive Relaxation

Progressive relaxation is based on the premise that the first step in relaxation is recognizing muscular tension when it occurs.

To accomplish this, ask your client to purposely tighten and hold a muscle, then to relax it slowly and completely, noticing the difference in the sensations that occur as they do so. Use a slow, soft voice as you describe what you want her to feel. As the muscle relaxes and tension is released, she should imagine it leaving the area, as a feeling of warmth and heaviness floats in. Use words and imagery that help to bring about a state of complete relaxation. Work your way through the entire body, first tightening and then relaxing all the major muscle groups, until the client has "let go" of tension in every area. End the session by having her lie quietly, feeling a relaxed heaviness and "sinking into the floor."

Popular Group Exercise Modes during Pregnancy

CHAPTER SIX

Teaching group exercise classes that integrate pregnant and non-pregnant exercisers has its challenges, including knowing who, if anyone, is pregnant, since many women will not "show" until well into their second trimester. Pre-exercise screening identifies the new exerciser, but it does not help to identify the regular exerciser who is newly pregnant. Consequently, it is important for you to announce periodically to your class the need to know about special conditions, such as pregnancies or injuries. Also, be available before and after class to talk with participants who may not feel comfortable making announcements or voicing concerns in front of the class.

Classes designed specifically for pregnant women have certain advantages over integrated classes. First, there is no problem identifying pregnant participants. Also, participants can be addressed as a group about relevant issues and monitored more readily for strain, discomfort, and fatigue. Perhaps one of the biggest advantages is that the pre-natal exercise class becomes a natural support group, where women can feel free to discuss feelings and share concerns and generally feel more "accepted" as their bodies change and grow. However, many women who have been participating in regular group exercise classes prior to their pregnancies will want to continue with them, and they should not be discouraged from doing so. This is especially true during early pregnancy when a favorite mode of exercise is not taught specifically for pregnant women (e.g., cycling).

Whether you are teaching pre-natal classes or integrated classes, communicate with pregnant participants about necessary modifications regarding an exercise, equipment usage, exercise intensity, and other issues. Be mindful of conditions such as hyperthermia, hypoglycemia, hypoxia, and musculoskeletal discomforts. If a pregnant participant finds any exercise awkward, uncomfortable, difficult, or embarrassing, have her stop, or give her a suitable modification.

Traditional Aerobics

Most women elect to discontinue high-impact aerobics during pregnancy due to associated discomforts. About 20% of those who continue with high-impact activities, like aerobics or running, have lower-abdominal discomfort or pelvic pressure (Clapp, 1998). The use of a maternity support belt may relieve this discomfort. However, the weight gain during mid- and late-pregnancy make high-impact aerobics a less-desirable form of exercise for most due to the increased biomechanical stress placed on the joints. Low-impact aerobics, on the other hand, can provide aerobic and strengthening benefits, and many pregnant women feel comfortable continuing with this activity through their third trimester.

Keeping music speed within recommended ranges, such as 120 to 140 bpm for low-impact aerobics, is important. Choreography should be relatively simple, keeping in mind that changes in a woman's center of gravity increase the balance and stability challenge of most low-impact movement patterns. Smooth flooring is important to prevent tripping. Avoid quick changes in direction and twisting movements, as they may stretch and cause discomfort in the ligaments supporting the uterus. Women experiencing this will complain of sharp pains in the abdominal area. Using good teaching techniques, such as allowing participants to learn new moves at half-speed, advance cueing to prepare for changes in movement direction or speed, and gradual "layering" of movements to build combinations, will allow pregnant exercisers to participate without feeling "clumsy" or "uncoordinated." If necessary, modify intensity by decreasing the range of motion used and by eliminating upper-body involvement.

Step Training

Although step training is a weight-bearing exercise, it is low-impact and, therefore, a favorite form of exercise during pregnancy. Early in pregnancy, most women who step train can continue at their pre-pregnancy step height. However, as body weight increases, the amount of oxygen required to lift oneself up onto the step increases as well. Consequently, it becomes necessary for most pregnant women to gradually lower the height of the step to achieve the same relative exercise intensity. Those who start at lower platform heights can eliminate the step altogether later in pregnancy and perform the same step patterns on the floor. Tape placed on the floor outlining the size and shape of a step will help participants continue with the rest of the class at an appropriate intensity.

While stepping, advise participants to lean the whole body slightly forward from the hips. This will help them to avoid an exaggerated sway-back posture. Always provide modifications for pregnant women integrated into a regular step class. Propulsive moves will be difficult for

many, so provide other options. Simplified choreography that involves few lateral movements is recommended. Consider pregnant women's altered balance when choosing movement patterns. A good reason to keep choreography simple is that in the later stages of pregnancy, it is difficult for women to see the step when looking down because their bellies are in the way.

Pregnant women often experience foot discomfort due to weight gain edema, causing increased pressure in the foot. Wearing a slightly larger shoe size with good support can help, as can orthotics in some cases.

Group Indoor Cycling

While outdoor cycling involves the risk of falling and injury, indoor cycling does not. In fact, because it is non-weightbearing, it is an activity that many women feel comfortable performing right up until their due date.

The changes in body size and shape that accompany pregnancy affect cycling biomechanics. The knees and hips rotate outward to accommodate the belly. Raising the handlebars to the most upright position allows pregnant women to sit in a slightly more vertical position and minimize the effects of the growing belly on pedaling mechanics. Unfortunately, this more upright position, coupled with the increased pelvic pressure from the baby, may contribute to more saddle discomfort. Padded seat covers and/or wider, female saddles will increase comfort. Some women find that late in pregnancy the pelvic pressure is too uncomfortable to continue cycling, while others have no problem. As long as women are comfortable and otherwise healthy, there is no reason to limit indoor cycling to a particular point in pregnancy.

Pregnant women who experience swelling in their ankles and feet often find their feet are uncomfortable or go numb when riding with non-cycling shoes and pedals that use toe-straps that constrict the foot. Cleated, properly fitted cycling shoes eliminate this problem and prevent slippage of the foot on the pedal (Anthony, 1998).

Caution pregnant women in the second half of pregnancy against too many out-of-the-saddle drills, especially at light resistance or with less-than-ideal technique. The increase in body weight, which is largely concentrated anteriorly, tends to pull a rider forward when out of the saddle. This forward leaning can place more pressure on the knees and increase the rider's tendency to fully extend or "lock out" the knees, both of which increase the injury risk. A pregnant rider must be allowed, and even encouraged, to stay in the saddle whenever she prefers to (Anthony, 1998).

Riding indoors generally increases body temperature and sweat production more than riding outdoors, and more so than many other types of group exercise. This is because indoor riders are stationary and do not benefit from the evaporative air currents created by outdoor riding. Since the fetus' ability to regulate its body temperature is dependent upon the mother's body temperature, it is important to avoid overheating or dehydration. Therefore, fans or open windows are a must. In addition, advise pregnant women to drink before, during, and after a cycling class.

Indoor cycling classes often involve high-intensity exercise. Francis et al. (1999) found that a "typical" class elicited an average heart rate of 80% to 95% of maximum. While this intensity may be fine for some pregnant women who are accustomed to cycling at such vigorous levels, it may not be for others. Most pregnant women will need to decrease resistance and/or cadence to achieve the same cardiovascular overload as their pregnancy advances. Caution pregnant women against overexertion, and remind them throughout class to rate their perceived exertion. If pregnant riders experience prolonged fatigue the rest of the day rather than increased energy levels, advise them to slow their pace.

A 40-minute cycling class has been shown to burn between 318 and 587 calories (Francis, 1998). Many classes are 45 to 60 minutes long, which means this value could be even higher. A typical low-impact class, by comparison, burns about 150 to 250 calories. Pre- and post-exercise snacks are a must for pregnant women participating in vigorous indoor cycling classes.

Yoga

Yoga has become a popular form of exercise during pregnancy, with specially designed pre-natal yoga classes and videos now widely available. Some forms of yoga provide a mild, gentle workout that energizes while promoting relaxation, both of which benefit pregnant women. Many women feel that yoga helps them to more fully connect with the new life growing within them. Yoga coordinates movement with breathing and self-awareness and promotes confidence in the capabilities of one's body. The breathing techniques used in yoga can also help prepare women for labor. Yogic breathing techniques can help women remain more calm and relaxed through the physical discomfort of labor instead of tensing up and bracing for each contraction (Carrico, 1997).

Some yoga postures require modification due to the increased size of the abdomen or instability about the pelvis. Be careful not to take movements to complete end range if there is pregnancy-induced laxity about the involved joint(s). Instruct women to stay within their comfort range and "listen to how their body feels," rather than trying to perform the movement perfectly. Changes in center of gravity will make some postures difficult due to balance issues. A chair, a wall, a step turned on end, or a body bar can help when balance is an issue. Keep a close eye on your students and, if a particular posture is uncomfortable or awkward, provide a modification or alternative. Generally speaking, deep twists, backbends, and most inversions are unsuitable for pregnant women. Avoid postures involving motionless standing or supine lying, as they may decrease cardiac output and fetal oxygen supply. Modify poses normally done on the belly by assuming a hands-and-knees or side-lying position. Use pillows as props for the back, hips, or knees to increase comfort for pregnant women.

Emphasize postures that strengthen the core and lower body and that release tension in the chest, shoulders, low back, neck, jaw, and face. Poses that are well-suited to the needs of pregnant women include the cat/cow (strengthens abdominals and stretches shortened low-back muscles) (see Figures 9 & 10, page 29), the downward facing dog (strengthens abdominals, arms, shoulders and stretches back, hamstrings) (Figure 20), the child's pose (relieves tension in low back and hips) (Figure 21), forward fold (stretches hamstrings, lengthens back) (see Figures 6b & c, page 27), and butterfly pose (stretches groin and hip areas) (Figure 22). The bridge pose, supported triangle, and squats are also good. Due to changes in a woman's center of gravity during pregnancy, free-standing squats may pose a balance problem for some. Variations to traditional squats are shown in Figure 23. Many variations and modifications of these and other traditional postures can be used as well. Since the aerobic

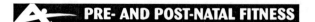

Figure 20

Downward facing dog. Begin on the hands and knees with the spine in a neutral position. Lift the knees and hips off the floor until the legs are extended and the body forms an inverted "V". Press the heels to the floor, keeping the legs slightly bent or straight and contracting the quadriceps. Look back at the feet, keeping the head and neck in line with the arms. Relax the neck. (Note: If this feels like too much of a stretch, the hands can be elevated onto a step.) Hold for several breaths, then lower the knees and move into the child's pose (see Figure 21, page 53).

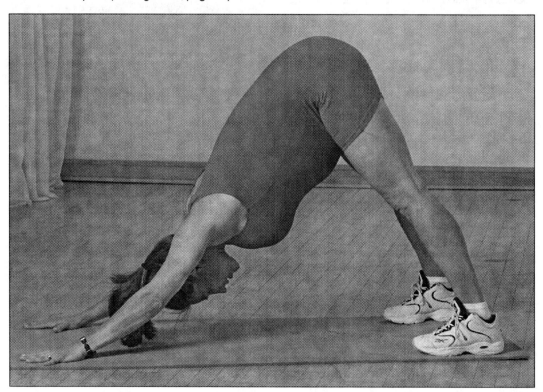

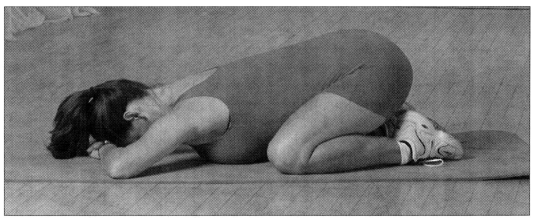

Figure 21
Child's pose. Transition from the downward facing dog position or begin on hands and knees. Move the knees wide apart to accommodate the belly and keep the toes together. Rest the hips back on the heels and allow the head to rest on the hands, keeping the elbows bent. Relax the muscles in the low back and allow them to lengthen.

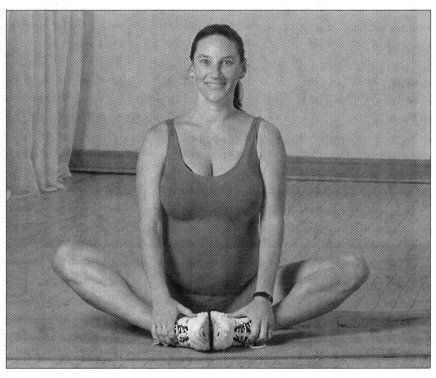

Figure 22
Butterfly pose. Sit with the knees bent and the soles of the feet pressed together. Do not round the lower back. Tuck the tailbone under and continue to press the feet together while letting the knees fall open to the sides. Lean forward slightly to increase the stretch if needed.

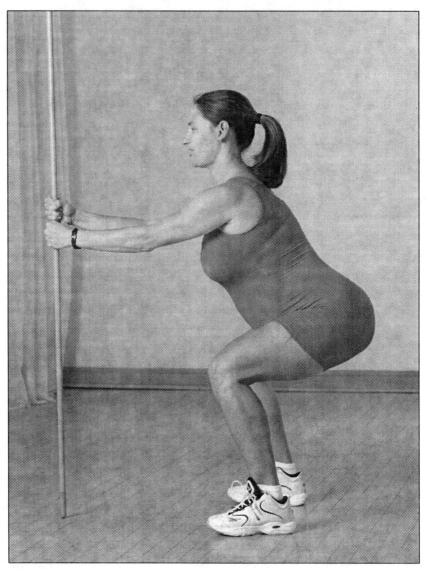

a.

Figure 23

Modifications to the basic squat. Additional support may be necessary during pregnancy due to the change in a woman's center of gravity and the associated balance issues.

a. A dowel or body bar can be used as a prop to aid with balance. A step turned on its end also works well. Take care to maintain neutral alignment through the pelvis and low back.

b. **Wall squat with the stability ball**. Begin with the ball placed between the low back and the wall and the feet comfortably away from the wall and hip-width apart.

c. **Wall squat with the stability ball.** Slowly lower into a squat position while rolling the ball down the wall. Return to the starting position by straightening the legs and rolling the ball back up the wall.

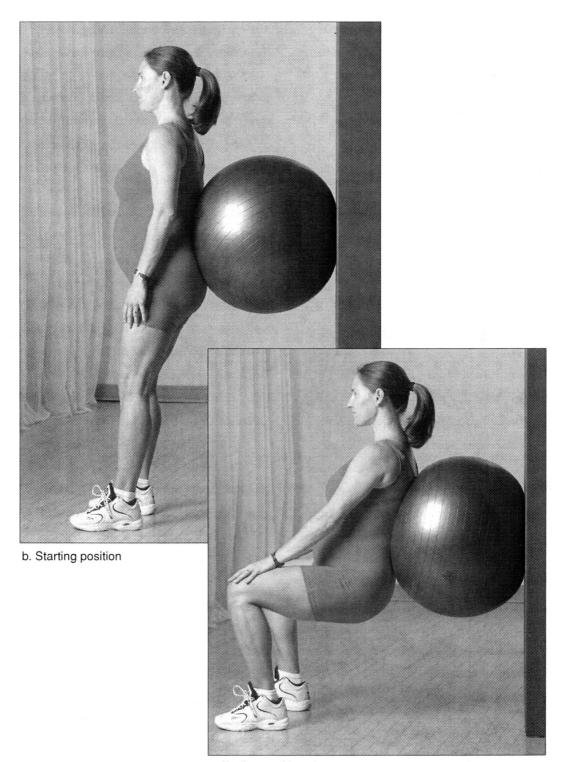

b. Starting position

c. Ending position

benefits of yoga are minimal, remind participants to also incorporate walking, bike riding,
or other low-impact cardiovascular exercise into
their routine three to four days per week.

Aquatic Exercise

Water activities are a favorite among
pregnant women. The water's
buoyancy provides comfort by
supporting a pregnant woman's body weight and
eliminating balance deficits caused by shifts in
their center of gravity. Water exercise is easier
on the musculoskeletal system than weightbearing land exercise, due to the reduced stress
placed on the joints and ligaments. The water
can provide relief for the muscles that are
shortened and fatigued from bearing the
mechanical stress of pregnancy, while allowing
women to enjoy exercising with a wonderful,
weightless feeling. The buoyancy of water also
lifts the weight of the uterus off the bladder and
relieves pressure in the pelvic area. Women in
late pregnancy who cannot continue with a land-
based exercise program due to back or pelvic
discomfort are often able to exercise with ease in
the water.

The hydrostatic pressure present in an aquatic
environment can also lessen fluid retention and
swelling, which are common complaints during
pregnancy. Standing in a vertical position in 5
feet of water creates a hydrostatic pressure on
the body that exceeds diastolic pressure, thereby
assisting circulation and reducing swelling all

over the body (Lawton and Coberly, 2000).
Swimming, or other water exercise in the prone
position, also facilitates blood flow to the uterus
by redistributing the weight of the uterus away
from the inferior vena cava and the aorta
(Anthony, 2000). The hydrostatic effects of the
water are also associated with a smaller plasma
volume decrease than occurs during exercise on
land, which may result in better maintenance of
uterine and placental blood flow.

Aquatic exercise has the added benefit of
aiding thermoregulation, provided the water
temperature is not too warm. Most women will
feel comfortably cool exercising in water that is
between 78° and 85°F (26° to 29°C).
Discourage exercise in water that is too warm
(e.g., hot tubs) due to the potential thermal stress
on the fetus.

Pregnant women can exercise in the supine
position in water, as the hydrostatic effects
eliminate problems with supine hypotensive
syndrome. Reduce the intensity of strengthening
exercises for hip adductors and abductors for
those with feelings of instability in the pelvis.
Likewise, use caution with forceful frog or whip
kicks in susceptible individuals. Traditional use
of a kickboard (kicking while prone with the
head held high) may amplify the already
exaggerated lordotic curve associated with
pregnancy, furthering fatigue in the chronically
shortened and tightened low-back muscles.
Individual comfort and symptoms should
determine kickboard use. Pregnant swimmers

often enjoy using pull buoys (flotation devices for the legs), because they keep the legs and abdomen in a more horizontal position, rather than sinking deeper into the water as lower-body density increases.

Aquatic exercise instructors will find it relatively easy to "mainstream" pregnant exercisers into traditional classes, and only a few modifications usually need to be made. To maintain or improve aerobic fitness and endurance for labor, water exercise for pregnant women should include a cardio-vascular exercise segment of 20 to 30 minutes that uses large muscle groups in a dynamic, rhythmic fashion and is vigorous enough to elicit an RPE of 6 to 7.

Water provides resistance 12 to 15 times that of air (Di Prampero, 1974). This makes it possible to target both cardiovascular and muscular endurance exercise at the same time (Sanders, 2001). Examples include forward and backward jogging, jumping jacks, and scissor movements with the arms and legs. Strengthening exercises using the water as resistance will help to maintain functional capacity and prepare women for caring for their newborn. Advise women to perform stretching exercises for the low back and chest, and strengthening exercises for the abdominals and upper back, to counterbalance the postural stresses of pregnancy.

Group Strength Training

Strength training is a beneficial and safe activity during a normal, uncomplicated pregnancy if the standard safe practices of weightlifting are adhered to closely. Pregnant women who strength train can maintain or increase muscular strength and endurance, maintain muscle tone, improve posture, and reduce low-back pain. Regular strength training may offset the effects of pregnancy on ligamentous laxity and protect relaxed joint structures (Clapp, 1998). Lastly, strength training may help reduce the time needed to resume activities of daily life without undue fatigue in the postpartum period.

Free weights, balls, and tubing can all be used. Group strength training instructors must give close and constant attention to pregnant partic-ipants to make sure they stay in control of the weight and use slow, appropriate speeds and proper exercise technique. It is also extremely important for pregnant women to avoid the Valsalva maneuver (breath holding, or forced expiration against a closed glottis) when lifting to avoid changes in intra-abdominal pressure that could decrease oxygen supply to the fetus. Frequent reminders to "exhale on the effort" are helpful. Prolonged standing should also be avoided, as this has been shown to decrease fetal blood supply more than supine exercise. Structure your class to include frequent positional changes.

Base exercise selection on counterbalancing the biomechanical stresses of pregnancy and preparing for the physical demands women will face as new moms. Typically, new mothers spend much of their time carrying, lifting, nursing, and holding the new baby. These activities put the spine in forward flexed postures for extended amounts of time and can contribute to upper- and lower-back pain and injury. The emphasis during pre-natal training should be to develop the necessary muscular strength and endurance to ward off these chronic aches and pains common in new moms.

Exercises should focus on overall upper-body strength, with special attention given to the muscles of the upper back, which are prone to "stretch weakness" in the pre- and post-natal periods due to the increased gravitational pull of the enlarging breasts. Seated bilateral external shoulder rotation (with tubing) and scapular retraction on the stability ball are examples of effective upper-back exercises during pregnancy (Figures 24 & 25). Core stability, lower-body strength and endurance, and upper-body strength are also important considerations.

Repetitions and load should be determined by exercise history, state of pregnancy, motivation, and other variables. Women who have been participating in group strength training prior to becoming pregnant may be able to maintain their usual routine well into their second trimester, but several modifications become necessary as pregnancy advances. Familiarize

yourself with the amount of weight your participants use for each exercise early in their pregnancy, and give them "permission" to decrease it gradually if they are uncomfortable or if their technique is compromised as their pregnancy advances. Exercises that use body weight as resistance (e.g., squats, lunges) will quickly become more difficult as body weight increases, and it may be appropriate to eliminate external weight altogether. If balance becomes an issue, use external support (e.g., bar, wall, chair). Some exercises, such as push-ups, will need to be eliminated for most women as pregnancy advances. The gravitational strain on the low back and abdominal structures and the increase in body weight make push-ups a poor exercise choice, and more suitable alternatives can be provided. A wall push-up or seated chest press with tubing are good options. Offer alternatives to exercises that place women in a supine position after the first trimester due to the risk of supine hypotensive syndrome, and slowly change from lying and seated exercises to standing exercises to reduce the possibility of orthostatic hypotension.

Depending on the exercise being performed, different positions may be preferable during pregnancy. While lying supine is not recommended, standing exercises may also pose unique challenges to pregnant women in group strength training classes. As pregnancy advances, the growth of the baby makes maintaining a neutral spine and pelvis

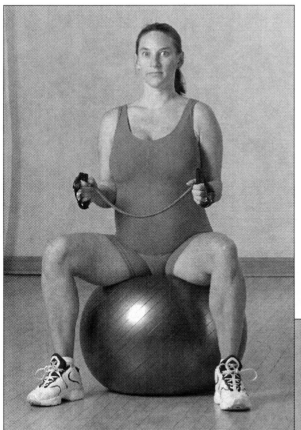

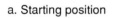
a. Starting position

Figure 24
Seated bilateral external rotation and scapular retraction.

a. Seated on a stability ball or bench, hold a shortened piece of tubing in both hands with the arms at the sides and flexed to 90° at the elbows.

b. Simultaneously pull both forearms back, keeping the upper arms at the sides and pulling the shoulder blades down and together. Release slowly, return to the starting position, and repeat.

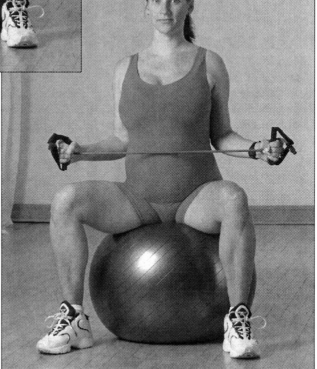

b. Ending position

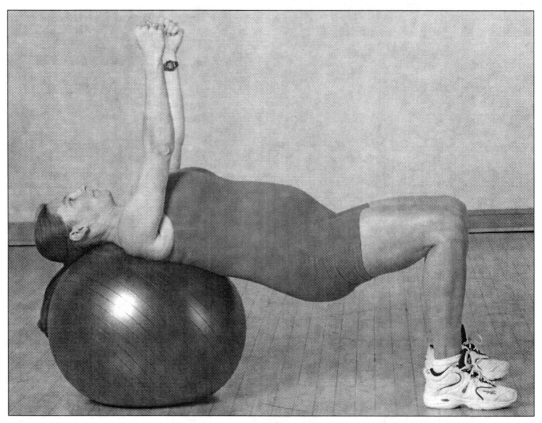

Figure 25
Scapular retraction on the stability ball. Position the body on the ball so the upper back, neck, and head are relaxed and supported. Feet are hip-width apart and flat on the floor, and the hips are in a modified bridge position. Extend the arms vertically. Press the shoulder blades down into the ball, attempting to squeeze the shoulder blades together. Arm position should not change during the movement. Hold for two to three seconds, release, and repeat while maintaining the bridge position.

challenging, especially when standing. Pregnant exercisers are less able to stabilize their spine against the pull of their belly due to the elongated and weakened position of the abdominals. Avoid exercises that involve this stabilization challenge while loading the spine (e.g., standing overhead press) (Anthony, 2000; Artal, 2000). The size and position of the enlarging belly will also interfere with certain exercises (e.g., upright row or bent over row with barbell). Fortunately, numerous alternatives exist that can be used in these situations. Offer seated or kneeling alternatives to exercises normally done in a standing position for women in their second half of pregnancy (e.g., seated biceps curl versus standing) to decrease stress on the back. Most importantly, remain flexible, and provide exercise options that allow your pregnant participants to continue training as long as they wish.

Post-natal Exercise

CHAPTER SEVEN

Recovery from the Birth Process

The first six weeks after the birth of the baby are an intense time for new moms. First, they need to recover from what is often a physically exhausting labor and delivery process. Next, although a new baby is a "good" stress, it creates stress nonetheless, as moms make the necessary adjustments to their lives to make room for a new family member. The rest they really need at this time is generally hard to come by. Baby needs to be fed every three to four hours and, unfortunately, has no regard for traditional notions of waking versus sleeping hours!

Let women know that the priority of these first six weeks should be bonding with the baby and taking advantage of every opportunity to get necessary rest. How exercise fits into this picture will vary among individuals. Some women feel that finding time and energy to exercise during this period is just one more stressor, or they feel guilty about being away from the baby to exercise. Others find exercise to be just the mental and emotional break they need, providing them with "personal time" to relax and refocus. These women find time away from the baby spent exercising helps keep them from feeling overwhelmed or "out of control." These are the first symptoms of postpartum depression, which affects one in four first-time mothers. Returning to activity after pregnancy has been associated with a decrease in postpartum depression (Artal, 1992), but only if it is stress-relieving and not stress-provoking. For those who choose to resume exercise in these early weeks, the goal of exercise should be to help with relaxation, stress management, and emotional well-being. ACOG recommends that pre-pregnancy exercise routines be resumed gradually, based on a woman's physical capability. Vigorous exercise and goals of "getting my old body back" are premature at this time. Let your clients know that getting back in shape is a process that needs to be taken one step at a time; skipping steps will not make it happen any faster and may in fact result in setbacks. Exercise should cause no associated pain or increase in postpartum-related bleeding.

The first step in this process is resuming Kegel exercises as soon as possible, which is usually within the first 24 hours following delivery. Resuming Kegels will help the healing process of the pelvic floor, which has been traumatized by stretching and possibly by episiotomy or tears. (An episiotomy is an incision made between the vagina and the rectum to provide more room for delivery of the baby.) Rehabilitate the pelvic floor before initiating any strenuous abdominal exercise. Have pregnant clients perform transverse abdominal work (abdominal compression) and pelvic tilts early in the postpartum period. Scapular retraction and stretches for the chest are also important to counterbalance the hunched over postures of holding and feeding the baby.

The suggested time for return to exercise is after the postpartum doctor appointment, usually six weeks. Before this appointment (weeks two through five), encourage women to resume a gentle walking program. Initially, this should be nothing more than a 5- to 10-minute walk around the block, progressing gradually by adding about 5 minutes per week. Walking will help to tone and strengthen the muscles of the lower body and, to some extent, the torso. Have clients focus on good spinal alignment while walking to help strengthen important postural muscles that have weakened during pregnancy. Women who exercise during pregnancy and resume it early in the postpartum period have a shorter duration of urinary stress incontinence than those who do not (Morkved & Bo, 2000).

Resuming Exercise

As your clients return to exercise at about the six-week mark, perhaps the most difficult job for you is keeping them motivated in their exercise goals, while at the same time providing them with a reality check. Goals at this time are often unrealistic and can result in feelings of frustration ("Why isn't this working?"). The truth is, a return to pre-pregnancy body composition (not just body weight) will take nine months to a year in most cases. Your job is to help create an environment that discourages weight loss as the sole reason to exercise and leaves your postpartum clients feeling encouraged, uplifted, and invigorated. Remember that caring for an infant is a 24-hour-a-day, seven-day-a-week commitment. Lack of sleep, coupled with increased anxiety and tension, may affect not only the health and well-being of new mothers, but their relationship with the baby and other family members as well. Exercise should be comfortable, allowing new mothers time for self-care and time to master necessary coping skills.

Breast and Abdominal Support

Good breast support is key to comfort during postpartum exercise. Participants should wear a supportive exercise bra, or even wear two together if necessary. Breastfeeding women should not exercise with a breast abscess or with painful, engorged breasts. Some women may also feel that the lax abdominal wall needs support to prevent bouncing; tights or a pregnancy support belt can provide support and improve comfort.

Back Pain

Upper- and lower-back pain are common in the postpartum period, and postpartum classes need to address both. After delivery, the overstretched abdominal wall is loose and unsupportive to the low back. This weakness, combined with poor biomechanics while caring for the infant, can predispose new mothers to back pain. The muscles of the torso need to be retrained to effectively stabilize the spine. Upper-back pain is often caused by increased weight in the breasts from lactation, coupled with the forward rounded postures used when holding, feeding, and cuddling the baby. Lifting a car seat and pushing a stroller with handles that are too low can also contribute to the problem. Stretches for the chest, followed by scapular retraction and shoulder external rotation exercises, can help.

The following exercise sequence is an effective way to recondition the core musculature in postpartum women (Figures 26 to 29). Exercisers should first engage the pelvic floor and transverse abdominal muscles (hollowing). Abdominal bracing is then held while limb movements are added to provide progressive resistance to lumbar stabilization.

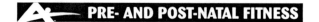

Figure 26

Abdominal bracing. First perform a Kegel exercise by "drawing up" the muscles
of the pelvic floor. Then, exhale while drawing the naval toward the backbone,
contracting the transverse abs. Maintain pelvic stabilization throughout the exercises shown in
Figures 26 to 29 by "bracing" with the abdominals in this way.

Abdominal bracing with arm movement.

a. While lying supine with the arms held straight up over the chest and the knees bent comfortably,
   find neutral spine and perform abdominal bracing. Slowly lower one arm straight back while
   lowering the other arm to the side of the body. Breathe evenly and keep the movement even and
   steady while stabilizing the trunk and pelvis.
b. Alternate the right and left arms while maintaining the alignment of the pelvis. Do not allow the
   lower back to arch.

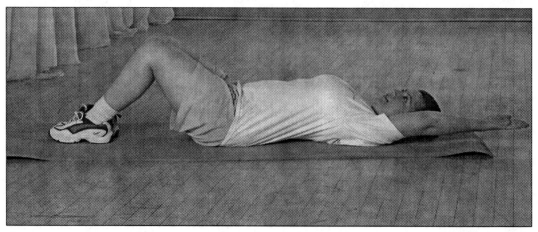

a.

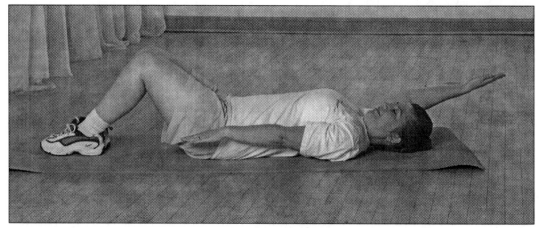

b.

Figure 27
Abdominal bracing with arm movement and legs extended. Perform abdominal bracing and arm movements as described in Figure 26 while keeping the legs extended. Maintaining a neutral pelvis is more challenging with the legs extended.

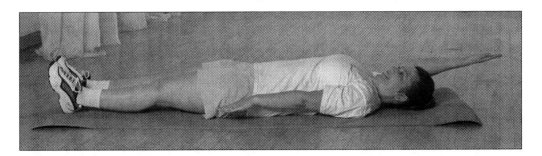

Figure 28
Abdominal bracing with double heel slide.
a. Lying supine with the abdominals tightened (abdominal hollowing) and low-back neutral, bend the knees and lift the toes off the ground.
b. Slowly extend both legs by sliding the heels away from the body while keeping the abdominals tight and the lower back pressed to the floor. Then slowly pull the heels back in toward the body in the same way. (Note: If this movement is too difficult, participants may find it easier to extend one leg at a time.)

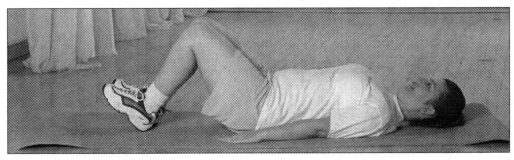

a.

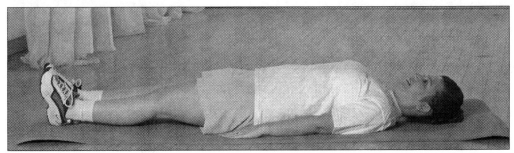

b.

Figure 29
Abdominal bracing with double toe taps.
a. From a starting position of lying supine with bent knees, feet on the floor, and abdominals "braced," lift the feet off the floor to create a 90° angle at the hips.
b. Exhale while slowly lowering both feet to tap the floor and return to the starting position. Do not allow the pelvis to tilt anteriorly; use the abdominals to stabilize the pelvis against any movement. (Note: If this movement is too difficult, participants may find it easier to lower one foot at a time.)

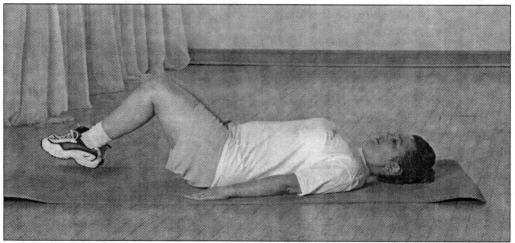

a.

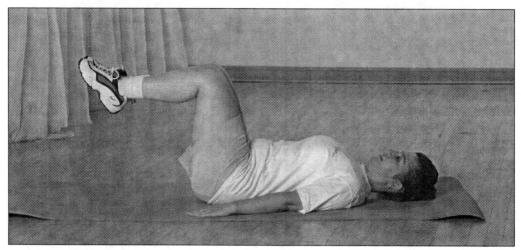

b.

Diastasi Recti

Further separation of a diastasis recti is of less concern postpartum than during pregnancy because the mechanical stress on the abdominals (the baby) is no longer exerting force against them. However, a significant diastasis is still to be noted: Its presence is evidence of an impaired core stabilization system. All women will exhibit some degree of separation, but if it is three fingers or more in width, special care and attention are warranted and proper exercise progressions must be employed (Table 9). It is a good idea to limit abdominal exercise to isometric transverse abdominal work and pelvic tilts until the gap has narrowed to two finger widths or less.

Resuming Exercise After Caesarean Delivery

Women who have cesarean sections have had their babies delivered surgically through the wall of the uterus and abdomen instead of through the vagina. Caesarean section, also called C-section, is a major abdominal surgery and, as such, results in pain and tenderness in the abdomen for some time, as well as considerable fatigue. However, the norm today is for mothers who deliver by C-section to be discharged by the third day; in years past, the hospital stay for these women was up to two weeks. Doctors now realize that prolonged bed rest for these individuals slows the rehabilitative process, not unlike in heart attack patients. Walking as soon as possible helps to minimize muscle wasting, increases circulation, and speeds the healing process. Even during the first 24 to 48 hours after surgery, gentle range-of-motion exercises can be performed in bed. Also encourage rising to a standing position, although pain may make it difficult to stand with good posture. Deep breathing, abdominal compression, and Kegel exercises can also be resumed early in the rehabilitation process.

Most Caesarean incisions do not actually cut the abdominal muscles; the incision is made through the skin and the doctor pushes aside the muscles to open the uterus and deliver the baby. Due to the advances in surgical procedures, many women who have undergone

---

Table 9

Sample Training Progression for Postpartum Closure of Diastasis and Abdominal Reconditioning

1. Kegel exercise
2. Kegel with abdominal compression or hollowing (transverse abs)
3. Kegel, abdominal hollowing; maintain while performing pelvic tilts
4. Kegel, abdominal hollowing; maintain while performing partial curl-ups
5. Maintain above sequence, layering on other abdominal exercises (e.g., crunches, reverse crunches)

C-section are ready to resume intermittent walking or other gentle forms of exercise by two weeks post-partum. During this time, the degree of discomfort, fatigue, and motivation will determine their activity levels. Vigorous exercise is to be avoided; the goal is to encourage the healing process by performing rehabilitative exercises and by getting adequate rest for the recovery process. Postpone re-entry into a structured exercise program until a doctor's clearance has been obtained after the six-week check-up. Women who have had C-sections may then participate in the same postpartum exercise programs as women who have had vaginal births, with similar guidelines. Any activity causing pain should be avoided. While most incisions from C-section heal without complications, some may develop scar tissue or adhesions that cause discomfort months after the surgery. Massage can sometimes be of help in these cases.

Breastfeeding and Exercise

Research has shown that regular, sustained, moderate-to-high intensity exercise does not impair the quality or quantity of breast milk (Dewey, 1998; Fly & Uhlin, 1998; McCrory, 2000). There are a small number of cases of exercise-induced increases in the lactic acid concentration of breast milk resulting in decreased infant suckling, due to a sour taste (Wallace, 1993). However, this problem was only encountered when the exercise was intense enough to result in lactic acid accumulation in the muscles (e.g., anaerobic interval training). Typically, aerobic workouts have not been shown to affect infant suckling behavior. Feeding the baby prior to exercise should negate any potential problem, as any lactic acid that does accumulate in the breast milk should clear by 30 to 60 minutes post-exercise. As long as infant suckling behavior is normal, neither high-intensity exercise nor lactic acid accumulation pose any risk to mom or baby.

Other research has examined the effect of exercise on immunoglobulin A (IgA), a major immune defense component, and found that breast milk IgA levels were slightly reduced after exercise. Whether this reduction could compromise infant health is not known, but the investigators' recommendation was to breastfeed before exercise to eliminate the risk of any potential adverse effects (Gregory et al., 1997). Research investigating the effects of exercise on the mineral content of breast milk found no significant effect (Fly & Uhlin, 1998).

Breastfeeding requires intake of an additional 300 to 500 calories per day. Most breastfeeding women spontaneously increase their caloric intake to the necessary amount. If infant weight gain is normal (approximately ¼ to ½ pound per week), maternal caloric intake is generally adequate. A recent study of postpartum women found that a moderate energy deficit of 35%, achieved by a combination of dieting and exercise, results in moderate weight loss that preserves lean mass and does not adversely affect lactation (Dewey, 1998). While eating enough calories is not usually a problem, adequate fluid intake often is. Breastfeeding requires roughly two additional quarts of water per day, a 30% increase in fluid intake, and exercise increases this need. Avoiding dehydration is very important in breastfeeding women, as it can decrease the volume of milk produced for the baby. You can help by reminding clients to drink at least 6 to 8 ounces of water for every 15 to 20 minutes of exercise and to grab a big glass of water every time they nurse their baby. Clapp (1998) recommends women monitor hydration status by noting the color of their urine—the paler, the better. If the baby seems content after feeding and not cranky, and wets five to six diapers a day, hydration is probably adequate.

Mother and Baby Classes

"**M**ommy and Me" classes are designed so women can engage in postpartum exercise while their

Table 10
Key Points for Postpartum Exercise
- Keep fluid intake high (urine should be pale).
- Wear good breast support.
- Stop exercise if there is any pain or increase in bleeding.
- Exercise should not be so vigorous as to create additional fatigue.
- Start slowly and increase gradually but steadily.

babies are in a front carrier, or close by in the same room. Classes are typically taught with the infants in the front carriers for the aerobic segment and in the front carriers or on the floor for the strength segment. Most front carriers do provide head support for the babies, but many of the exercises done without the carrier will require that the babies are old enough to hold their heads up. A variety of exercises can be done that involve interacting with the babies, sometimes even using them as a form of resistance (Figures 30 to 38). Women enjoy the social interaction with their babies as well as other moms. These classes also provide new moms an opportunity to share the joys and frustrations of motherhood, without leaving their babies. And, as the babies grow bigger and heavier, there is a natural progression in workout intensity.

Mother and baby classes have advantages to the fitness facility as well. These classes are usually held at off-peak traffic times, when the group exercise room is not in use. The classes can fill downtime on the schedule and generate additional revenue and additional members. Another plus is that no childcare staffing is needed. Stroller classes, held outdoors where weather permits, are an alternative if space is a problem.

As babies grow, postpartum women inevitably "graduate" from these classes and return to regular group exercise, so a steady stream of new participants is necessary to keep the program alive. Word of mouth is the best advertising, so be sure to send the women attending your pre-natal classes a card congratulating them on the births of their babies and informing them of your postpartum mother and baby class. Also, pediatricians who are looking to grow their practices can often be enticed to give short talks on childcare issues to your classes, welcoming an opportunity to leave their cards for potential patients or to lecture in exchange for a free membership. These physicians can become a valuable referral source and help your program succeed.

Figure 30
Biceps curl with baby.
a. Stand with feet hip-width apart, knees soft, abdominals engaged, shoulders retracted, and hands comfortably under the baby.
b. Slowly lift the baby up by flexing the elbows and performing a biceps curl.

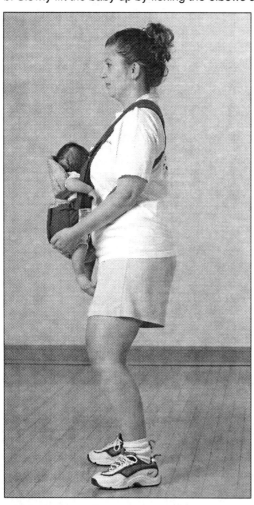

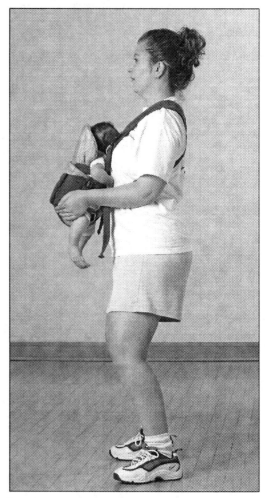

a.

b.

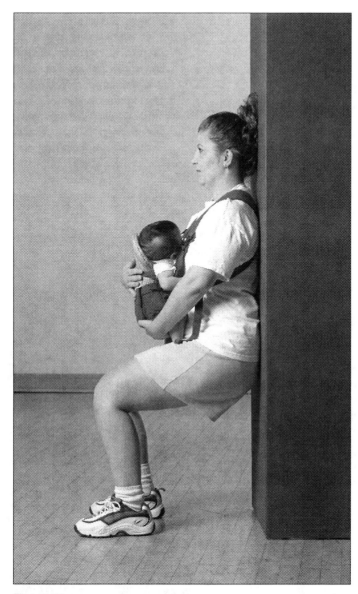

Figure 31
Wall squat with baby. The weight of the baby adds resistance to the traditional wall squat. Standing with the back against a wall and the feet about 1½ feet from the wall, slide down into a squat position. Hold for three to five seconds, release, and then return to the standing position.

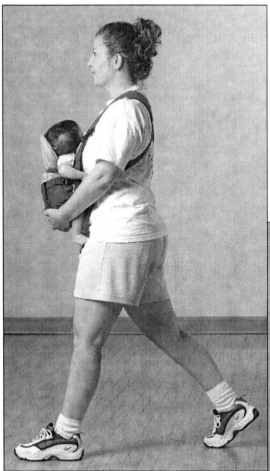

a. Starting position

Figure 32
Stationary lunge with baby.
Begin in a lunge position with knees soft, taking care to keep the eyes up, head lifted, and shoulders retracted. Lower the body, sinking most of the weight through the front hip and heel. Push straight up and return to the starting position. Do not allow the weight of the baby to pull the shoulders forward.

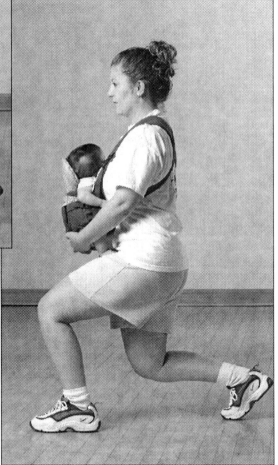

b. Ending position

Figure 33
Lat row with baby.
From a standing position with knees soft, hinge forward at the hips, maintaining the neutral curves of the spine. Hold the baby with the arms extended and one hand on the chest and the other on the stomach. Lift the baby up to the chest with the arms close to the sides and elbows pushing up. Lower the baby to the starting position and repeat.

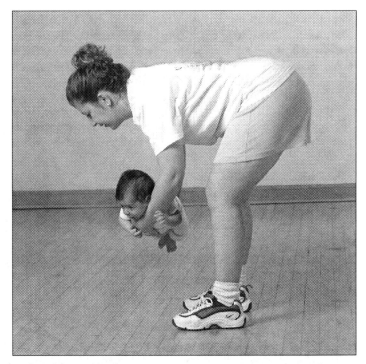

a. Starting position

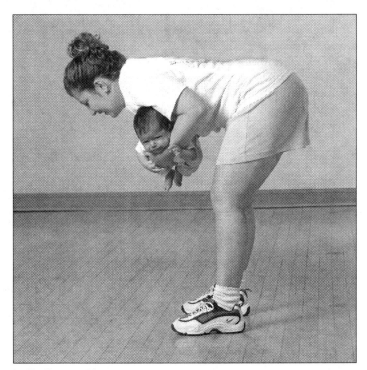

b. Ending position

Figure 34

Abdominal curl-up with baby. Lying supine with the knees bent, hold the baby against the thighs with the baby's head and back supported. Perform a Kegel exercise and abdominal hollowing. While maintaining the Kegel and abdominal hollowing, perform a partial curl-up while drawing the ribs toward the hips. Lower back to the floor, relax, and repeat.

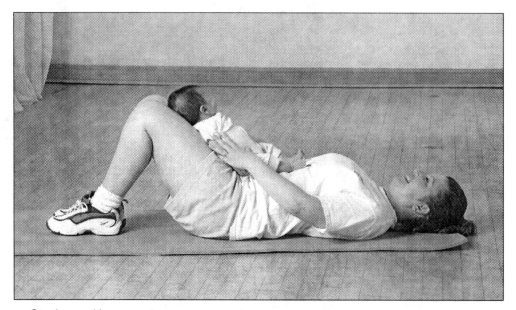

a. Starting position

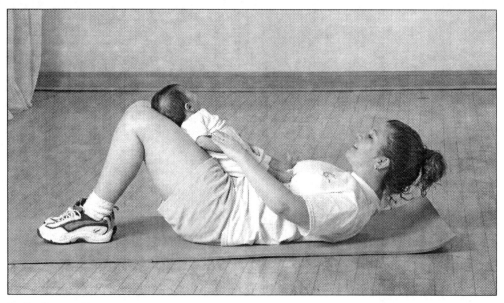

b. Ending position

Figure 35
Toe taps and abdominal bracing with baby. Begin by lying supine with knees and hips fixed at 90° and hold the baby over the chest. Perform Kegel exercise and abdominal compression (contract the transverse abdominis muscles). Maintain abdominal bracing while slowly lowering one leg at a time, tapping the foot on the floor, and slowly lifting it back to the starting position. Exhale while lowering each leg.

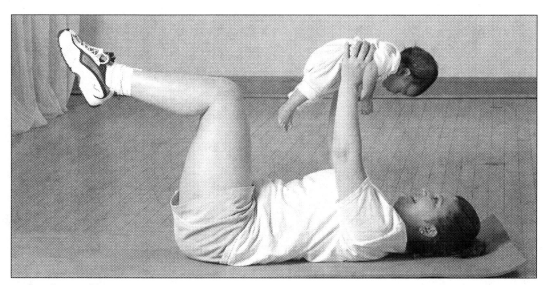

a. Starting position

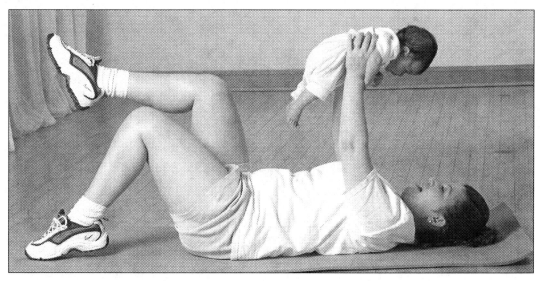

b. Ending position

Figure 36
Modified push-up with baby. Place the baby on his or her back and get into a modified push up position with the baby's feet between the mother's arms. Position the hands below the shoulders and keep the spine in neutral alignment. Lower the chest toward the baby, performing a modified push up.

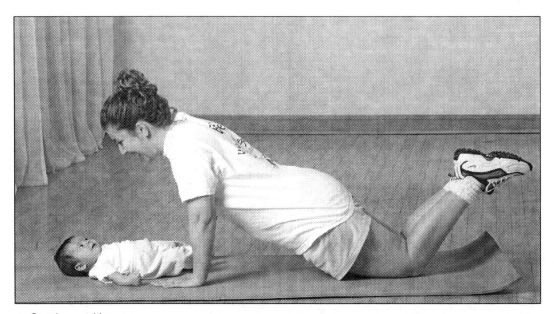

a. Starting position

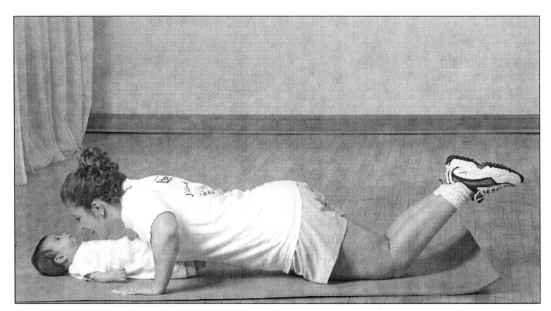

b. Ending position

Figure 37
Bridge with baby chest press. Begin in a supine position with knees bent, holding the baby on the chest. Perform and hold a Kegel exercise and abdominal hollowing. Extend the arms and press the baby up off the chest while bridging the hips and lower back off the floor. Avoid over-extending the hips and maintain neutral pelvis and spine throughout the exercise.

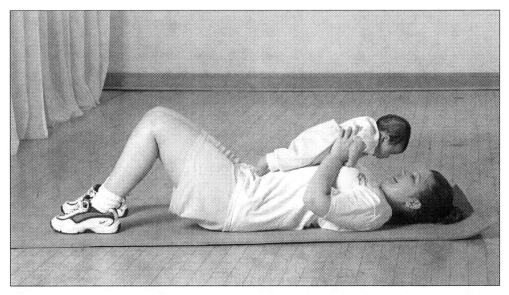

a. Starting position

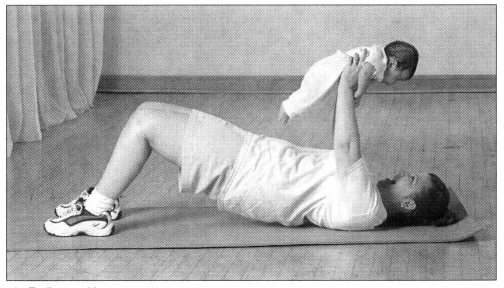

b. Ending position

Figure 38

Quadruped reciprocal reach. In an all-fours position, find neutral spinal alignment and place the baby with his or her feet between the arms. While maintaining a co-contraction of the back and abdominal muscles, slowly extend one arm and the opposite leg, hold momentarily, and lower slowly. Do not allow the opposing hip to drop as one leg lifts. Alternate sides. (Note: When teaching this exercise, begin by asking each participant to lift only the arm while maintaining neutral alignment. Once this is mastered, have them lift only the leg. Finally, have them try to extend both the arm and the opposing leg together.)

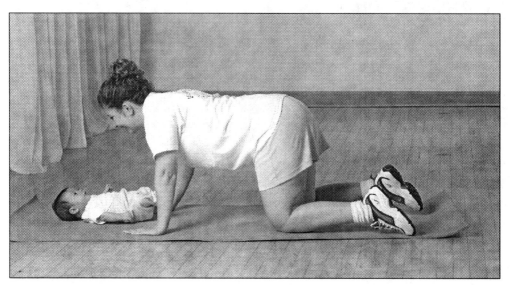

a.

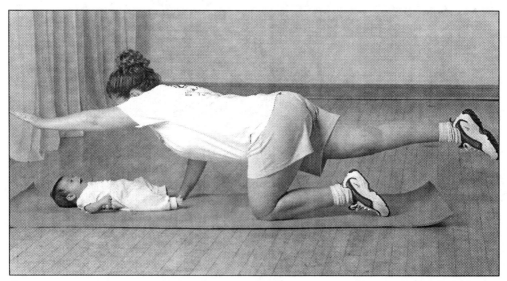

b.

A

abdominal bracing, 63, 64
 with arm movement, 64
 with arm movement and legs extended, 65
 with double heel slide, 65
 with double toe taps, 66
 toe taps and, with baby, 75

abdominal compression
 with Kegel exercise, 6, 39, 41,
  45, 67, 74, 75
 post-natal, 62, 63, 67, 74, 75
 pre-natal, 23, 38, 41

abdominal crunches, 24

abdominal curl-up
 with baby, 74
 post-natal, 67
 in semirecumbent position, 22

abdominal exercise
 and diastasis recti, 67
 in pre-natal group classes, 37–45

abdominal support, postpartum, 63

adduction/abduction machines, 25

adhesions, 68

advertising, mother and baby classes, 70

aerobic exercise
 absolute and relative contraindications
  to during pregnancy, 6
 and decrease in muscle cramps, 33
 high-impact, 48
 traditional, 48–49

American College of Obstetricians and
Gynecologists (ACOG)
 contraindications for exercise during
  pregnancy, 6
 on exercise intensity during
  pregnancy, 11, 35, 36
 guidelines for exercise during
  pregnancy, 2–3
 recommendation against exercising in
  supine position, 18

recommendations for post-natal
 exercise, 62

American College of Sports Medicine
(ACSM), 35

anemia, 10

aorta, 56

aquatic exercise, 25, 34, 56–57

athletes, and birth weight, 17

B

back pain
 postpartum, 63
 pre-natal, lower, 25–32, 39
 upper-back, 58, 63

balance, 8, 58

balls, 57

belly breathing, 38

belly-support system, 21, 48, 63

biceps curl with baby, 70

birth weight
 and exercise during pregnancy, 17
 and exercise frequency, 37
 and maternal food intake, 36

blood pooling, 10

blood volume, 10, 16, 34

body bar, 54

body temperature regulation
 and aquatic exercise, 56
 during pregnancy, 16

breastfeeding, 63, 68–69, 80

breast support, for post-natal exercise, 63, 69

breathing techniques, 46, 51

bridge pose, 51

bridge with baby chest press, 77

butterfly pose, 51, 53

C

Caesarean delivery
    incidence of, and exercise, 4
    resuming exercise after, 67–68

calories
    average requirements during breastfeeding, 68
    average requirements during pregnancy, 13
    burned in exercise, 36

carbohydrates
    fetal demand for, 13, 18
    utilization, 17

cardiac reserve, 10, 11

cardiovascular system
    changes during pregnancy, 10–11
    effect of changes on exercise, 11

carpal tunnel syndrome, 33–34

cat/cow stretch, 29, 51

center of gravity, changes in, 8, 48

chest press
    bridge, with baby, 77
    seated, with tubing, 58

child's pose, 51, 52, 53

choreography, 48

Clapp, J.F., III, 37, 69

clothing, 16

cramps, muscle, 33

crunches
    abdominal, 24
    incline with pelvic tilt on stability ball, 40

cueing, 45, 48

curl-ups, abdominal, 22, 67, 74

cycling, group indoor, 49–50

cycling shoes, 50

D

dehydration, 50, 69

diaphragm, 12

diastasis recti, 21–24, 67

dilutional anemia, 10

dizziness, 18, 38

downward facing dog, 51, 52

duration of exercise, 36

E

edema, 33, 56

emotional well-being, 62

endocrine system, 12

environmental temperature, 46

episiotomy, 62

estrogen, 12

exercise bra, 39, 63

F

fatigue, 3, 13, 39, 69

fetal hypoxia, 18, 38

fetal nutritional needs, 36

fetal risks
    carbohydrate utilization, 17
    hypothermia, 16–17
    supine hypotensive syndrome, 17–18

flooring, exercise, 48

flotation devices, 57

fluid intake. *See* hydration

fluid retention, 33, 56

American College of Obstetricians and Gynecologists. (1994). *ACOG Technical Bulletin.* Washington, D.C.: American College of Obstetricians and Gynecologists.

American College of Obstetricians and Gynecologists. (2002). *ACOG Committee Opinion: Exercise During Pregnancy and the Postpartum Period.* Washington, D.C.: American College of Obstetricians and Gynecologists.

American College of Sports Medicine. (2000, 1). *ACSM's Guidelines for Exercise Testing and Prescription,* 6th ed. Philadelphia: Lippincott, Williams & Wilkins.

American College of Sports Medicine. (2000, 2). *Current Comment: Exercise During Pregnancy.* Indianapolis: American College of Sports Medicine.

Anthony, L. (1995). Fit and pregnant. *IDEA Today*, Jan. 13, 1.

Anthony, L. (1998). Ask the experts: pregnancy and indoor cycling. *ACE Certified News,* 4, 5, 6.

Anthony, L. (1999). Ask the experts: diastasis recti. *ACE Certified News,* 5, 6, 8.

Anthony, L. (2000). Exercise and Pregnancy, in *ACE Group Fitness Instructor Manual.* San Diego, Cal.: American Council on Exercise.

Artal, R. (1992). Exercise and pregnancy. *Clinics in Sports Medicine,* 11, 2.

Artal, R. (2000). Exercise during pregnancy and the postpartum period. *ACOG Education Bulletin.*

Bungum, T.J. et al. (2000). Exercise during pregnancy and type of delivery in nulliparae. *Journal of Obstetrics, Gynecology and Neonatal Nursing*, May-June; 29, 3, 258–264.

Campbell, M.K. & Mottola, M.F. (2001). Recreational exercise and occupational activity during pregnancy and birth weight: a case-control study. *American Journal of Obstetrics and Gynecology,* February; 184, 3, 403–408.

Carrico, M. (1997). *Yoga Basics.* New York: Henry Holt and Company.

Clapp, J.F., III. (1991). The changing thermal response to endurance exercise during pregnancy. *American Journal of Obstetrics and Gynecology,* 178, 3, 594–599.

Clapp, J.F., III. (1998). *Exercising Through Your Pregnancy.* Champaign, Ill.: Human Kinetics.

Clapp, J.F., III et al. (1998). The one-year morphometric and neurodevelopment outcome of the offspring of women who continued to exercise regularly throughout pregnancy. *American Journal Obstetrics and Gynecology,* 178, 3, 594–599.

Clapp, J.F, III. et al. (2000). Beginning regular exercise in early pregnancy: effect on fetoplacental growth. *American Journal of Obstetrics and Gynecology,* December: 183, 6, 1484–1488.

Clapp, J.F., III & Little, K.D. (1995). Effect of recreational exercise on pregnancy weight gain and subcutaneous fat deposition. *Medicine & Science in Sport & Exercise*, 27, 2, 170–177.

Dewey, K.G. (1998). Effects of maternal caloric restriction and exercise during lactation. *Journal of Nutrition*, February; 128 (2 Suppl):386S–389S.

Devine, C.M., Bove, C.F., & Olson, C.M. (2000). Continuity and change in women's weight orientations and lifestyle through pregnancy and the postpartum period: the influence of life trajectories and transitional events. *Social Science and Medicine*, February; 50, 4, 567–582.

Di Prampero, P. et al. (1974). Energetics of swimming in man. *Journal of Applied Physiology*, 37, 1, 1–5.

Fly, A.D. & Uhlin, K.L. (1998). Major mineral concentrations in human milk do not change after maximal exercise testing. *American Journal of Clinical Nutrition,* August; 68, 2, 345–349.

Francis, P.R., Stavig Witucki, A., & Buono, M.J. (1999). Physiological response to a typical spinning session. *ACSM's Health and Fitness Journal,* Jan/Feb, 30–36.

Goodwin, A., Astbury, J., & McKeeken, J. (2000). Body image and psychological well being in pregnancy: A comparison of exercisers and non-exercisers. *Australia and New Zealand Journal of Obstetrics and Gynecology,* November; 40, 4, 442–447.

Gregory, R.L. et al. (1997). Effect of exercise on milk immunoglobulin A. *Medicine & Science in Sports & Exercise,* 29, 1596–1601.

Hall, C. & Brody, L. (1999). *Therapeutic Exercise: Moving Toward Function.* Philadelphia: Lippincott, Williams & Wilkins.

Hummel-Berry, K. (1990). Obstetric low back pain. *The Journal of Obstetric and Gynecologic Physical Therapy,* 14, 1, 10–13 & 14, 2, 9–11.

Koltyn, K.F. & Schultes, S.S. (1997). Psychological effects of an aerobic exercise session and a rest session during pregnancy. *Journal of Sports Medicine and Physical Fitness*, December; 37, 4, 287–291.

Kooperman, S. (1999). Moms in Motion, Evanston, Ill.: Sara's City Workout.

Lasater, J. (1994). Yoga for pregnancy. *Yoga Journal,* January-February; 3–11.

Lawton, R. & Coberly, M. (2000). Rehabilitation therapy: taking the plunge. *Orthopedic Technology Review,* 2, 11, 36, 48, 51.

McCrory, M.A. (2000). Aerobic exercise during lactation: safe, healthful, and compatible. *Journal of Human Lactation*, May; 16, 2, 95–98.

McMurray, R.G. et al. (1991). The thermoregulation of pregnant women during aerobic exercise in the water. *European Journal of Applied Physiology*, 61.

Morkved, S. & Bo, K. (2000). Effect of postpartum pelvic floor muscle training in prevention of urinary incontinence: a one-year follow up. *British Journal of Obstetrics and Gynecology*, August; 107, 8, 1022–1028.

Noble, E. (1995). *Essential Exercises for the Childbearing Year,* 4th ed. Boston: Houghton Mifflin Company.

Rath, J.D. et al. (2000). Low back pain during pregnancy: helping patients take control. *The*

Journal of Musculoskeletal Medicine, 17, 223–232.

Rubin, A. (1999). Exercise for timely childbirth. *The Physician and Sportsmedicine*, January; 27, 1, 27–28.

Sampselle, C.M. & Seng, J. (1999). Physical activity and postpartum well-being. *Journal of Obstetrics, Gynecology, and Neonatal Nursing*, January-February; 28,1, 41–49.

Sanders, M.E. (2001). Water exercise for seniors improves living on land. *IDEA Health and Fitness Source*, June, 19, 6.

Sternfeld, B., Sidney, S., & Eskenazi, B. (1992). Patterns of exercise during pregnancy and effects on pregnancy outcome. *Medicine & Science in Sports & Exercise,* 24, S170.

Wallace, J.P. (1993). Breast milk and exercise studies. *ACE Certified News,* 3, 6–8.

Wallace, J.P., Inbar, G., & Ernsthausen, K. (1994). Lactate concentrations in breast milk following maximal exercise and a typical workout. *Journal of Women's Health,* 3, 91–96.

Wilder, E. (1988). *Obstetric and Gynecologic Physical Therapy.* Edinburgh: Churchill Livingstone.

Wolfe, L.A., Brenner, I., & Mottola, M. (1994). Maternal exercise, fetal well-being, and pregnancy outcomes, *Exercise and Sports Science Reviews*, 22, 145–194.

Yeo, S. et al. (2000). Effect of exercise on blood pressure in pregnant women with a history of gestational hypertensive disorders. *Journal of Reproductive Medicine,* April; 45, 4, 293–298.

Zhang, J. & Savitz, D.A. (1996). Exercise during pregnancy among U.S. women. *Annals of Epidemiology*, 6, 1, 53–59.

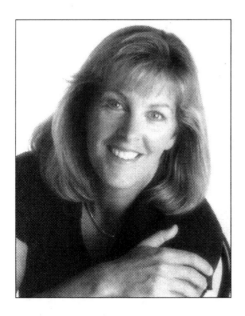

Lenita Anthony, M.S., is a clinical exercise physiologist and exercise specialist with 20 years of experience in group exercise and personal training. She is program coordinator at University of California, San Diego Extension in the Exercise Science & Fitness Instruction Certificate Program and an ACE-approved continuing education provider. A frequent industry presenter and author, Anthony is a Reebok University Master Trainer and program development team member and a contributing editor for IDEA publications. She is certified by ACSM as an Exercise Specialist.

ABOUT THE AUTHOR

91

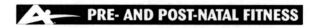

NOTES

NOTES